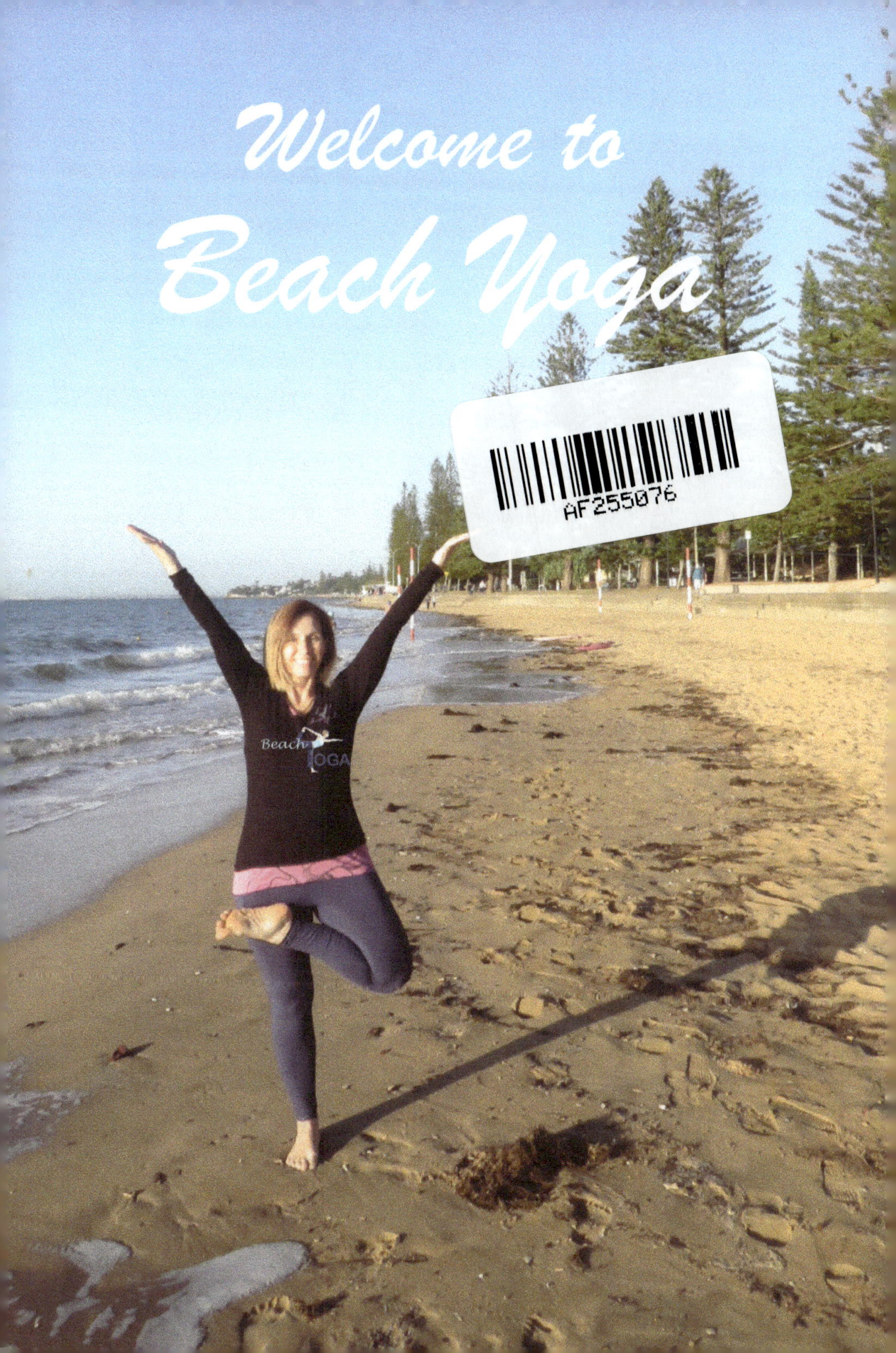

Welcome to
Beach Yoga
Beach
YOGA
AF255076

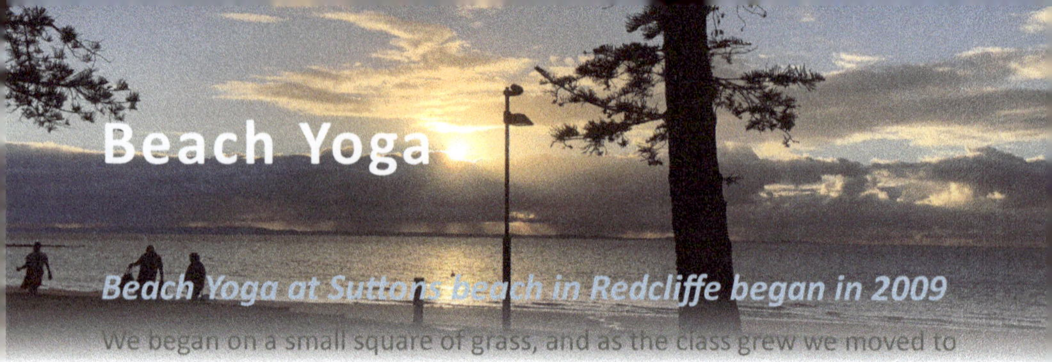

Beach Yoga

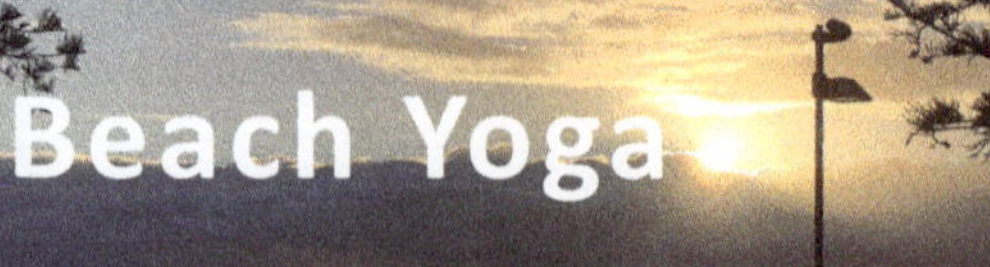

Beach Yoga at Suttons beach in Redcliffe began in 2009

We began on a small square of grass, and as the class grew we moved to wider and greener spaces on the southern lawn.

Every class is different, just like us. Every day the weather changes, just like us. We use the changing weather, landscape, and dynamic to plan each class. On warm sunny days we stretch and relax. On windy blustery mornings we strengthen and develop our balance and focus. During summer there are hundreds of runners, boot camps, athletes and families enjoying the park with us. In the winter it's just us, the sunrise, the ocean, and the birds.

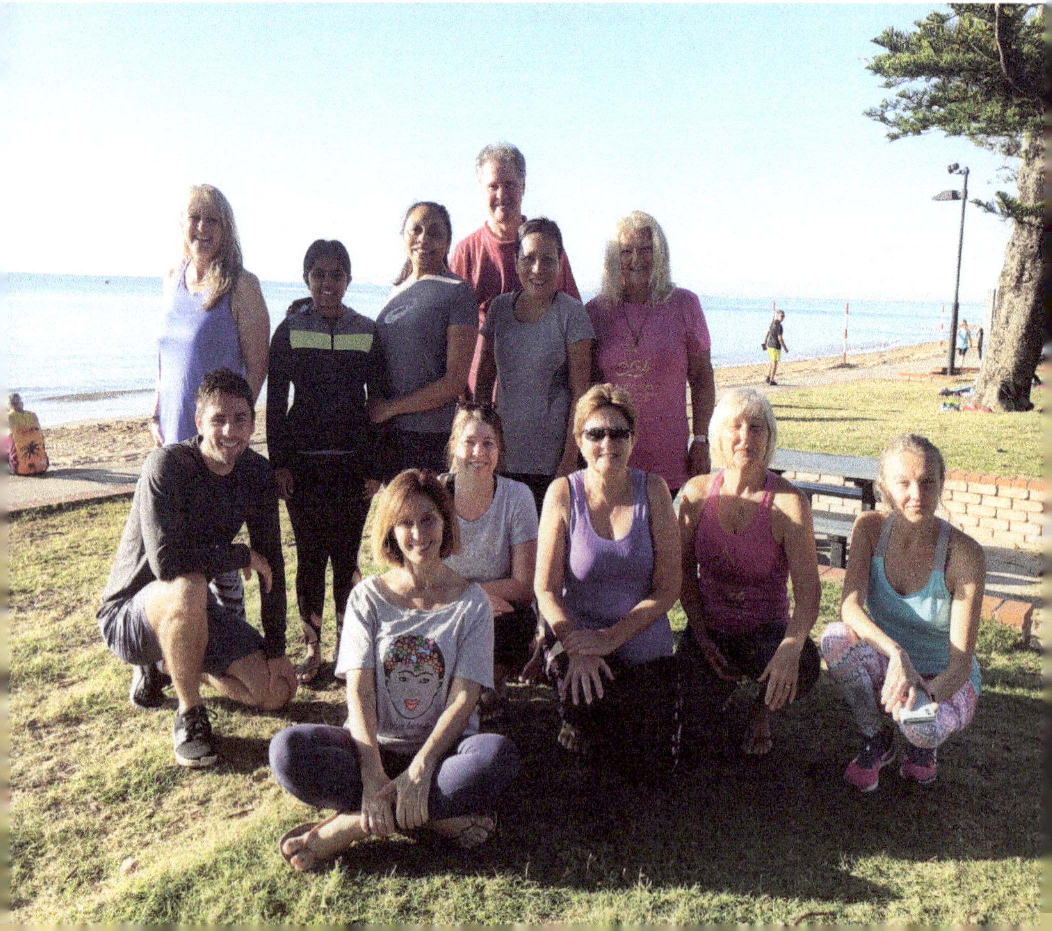

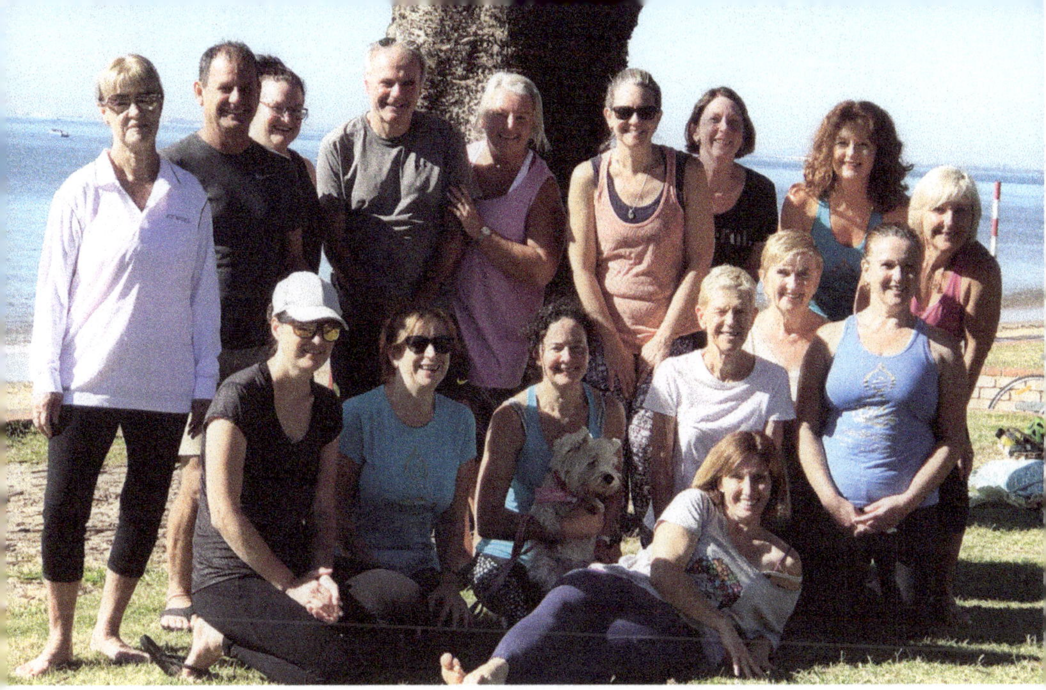

We've continued our classes through the Queensland floods, fires, and cyclones. When we can't be on the beach, we go to Monica's studio. During the 2020 lockdown we took our classes on live stream; Monica in her studio or at the beach, and her students watching from wherever they were.

We've formed lifelong friendships here under the trees. We've attended each other's milestones and supported each other through life's challenges.

I began *Beach Yoga* because I was burned out. I needed to work with something that could nurture me through. I found it in yoga. I found my breath, my strength, and my community. Yoga helped me physically, emotionally, and spiritually. My friends supported my business, my growth, and me. As a community we have grown with each other.

It was through *Beach Yoga* that I created my lifelong dream of becoming an artist and author. Since 2009 I've published several books and created many paintings.

I hope you enjoy our *Yoga Journal* and gain inspiration. We've been blessed with our yoga students and teachers. We hope you grow and blossom into yourself, because you are doing exactly what you need to be doing, just by being yourself.

Namaste Monica, Andreas, and the Beach Yoga team

about me

Name ____

Contact Details ________________________________

____

Important dates ________________________________

____

Things to remember _____________________________

____

Favourite colour _______________________________

Favourite food ________________________________

Favourite time of the day _________________________

Favourite yoga postures __________________________

Happy memory ________________________________

____

Goals for the next 5 years _________________________

____

Goals for the next 10 years ________________________

____

Goals for mind ________________________________

____

Goals for body ________________________________

____

Goals for spirit ________________________________

____

Goals for happiness _____________________________

____

My best friends ________________________________

____

A happy childhood memory

What I appreciate about myself

What I appreciate about my family

What I appreciate about my friends

Something I really want to do

Something I'm going to change this month

Something I'm going to change this year

Something I'm really good at

Something I'm proud of

A secret skill I have

What makes me feel loved

A charity I support

My commitment to loving myself more is to

Some ways to help me love myself more are to

One way I give back is to

My Ideal life

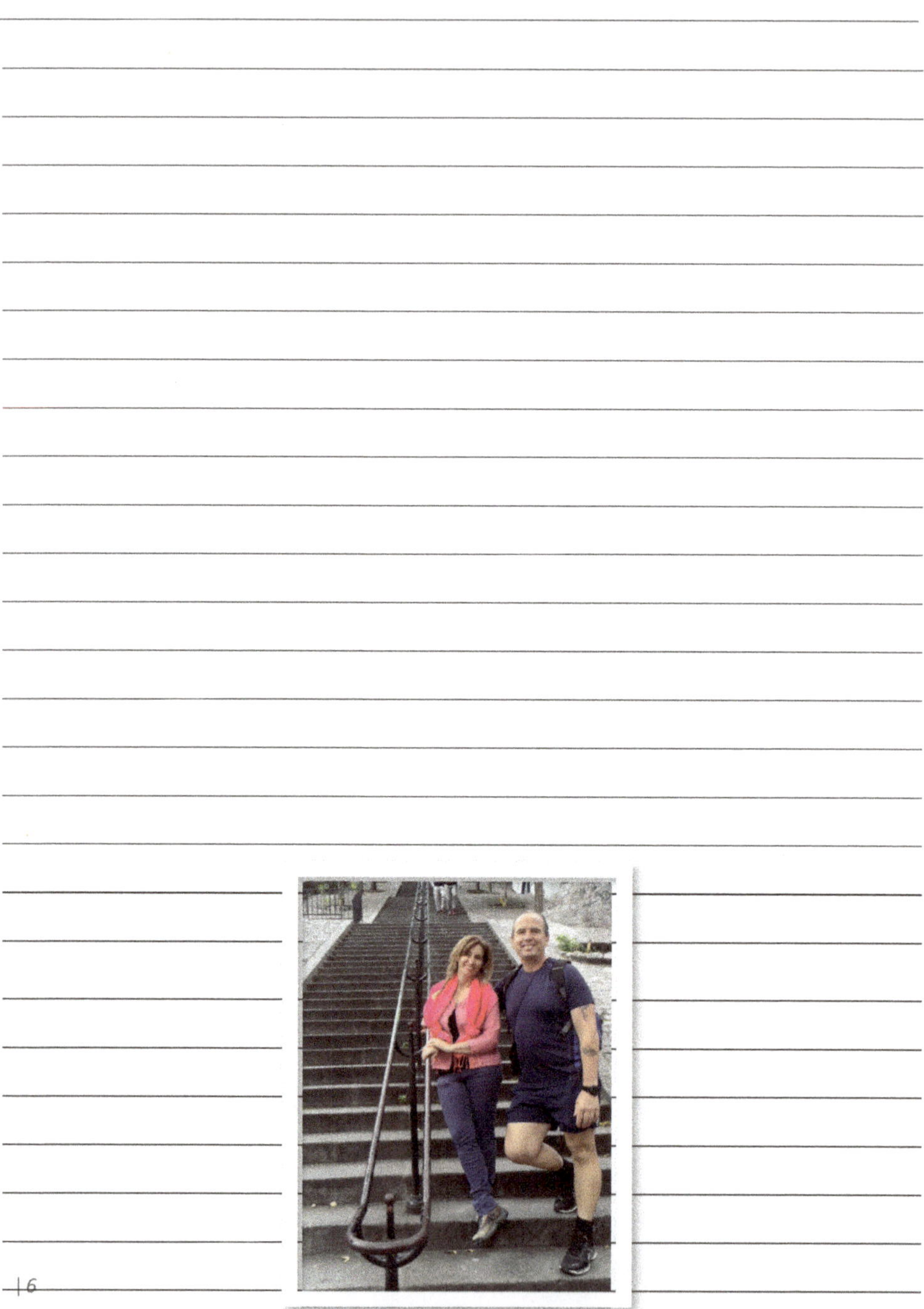

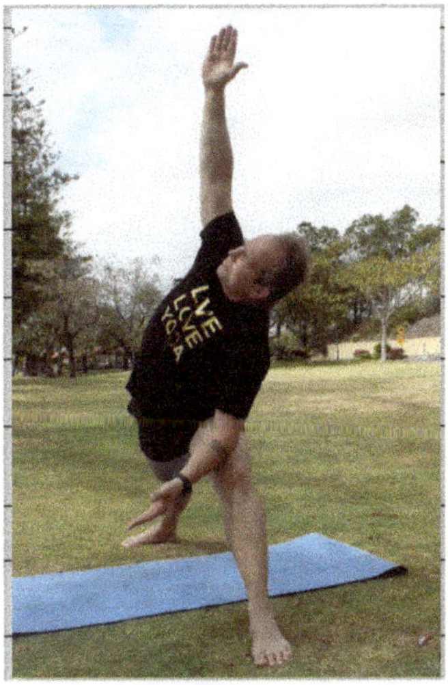

positive
AFFIRMATION

I can have, do, or be whatever I desire

I believe in myself

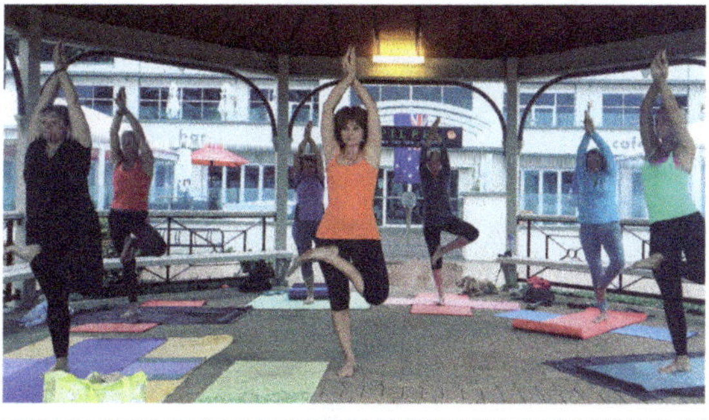

positive
AFFIRMATION

When I let go of resistance, all of my desires come to me

My yoga goals

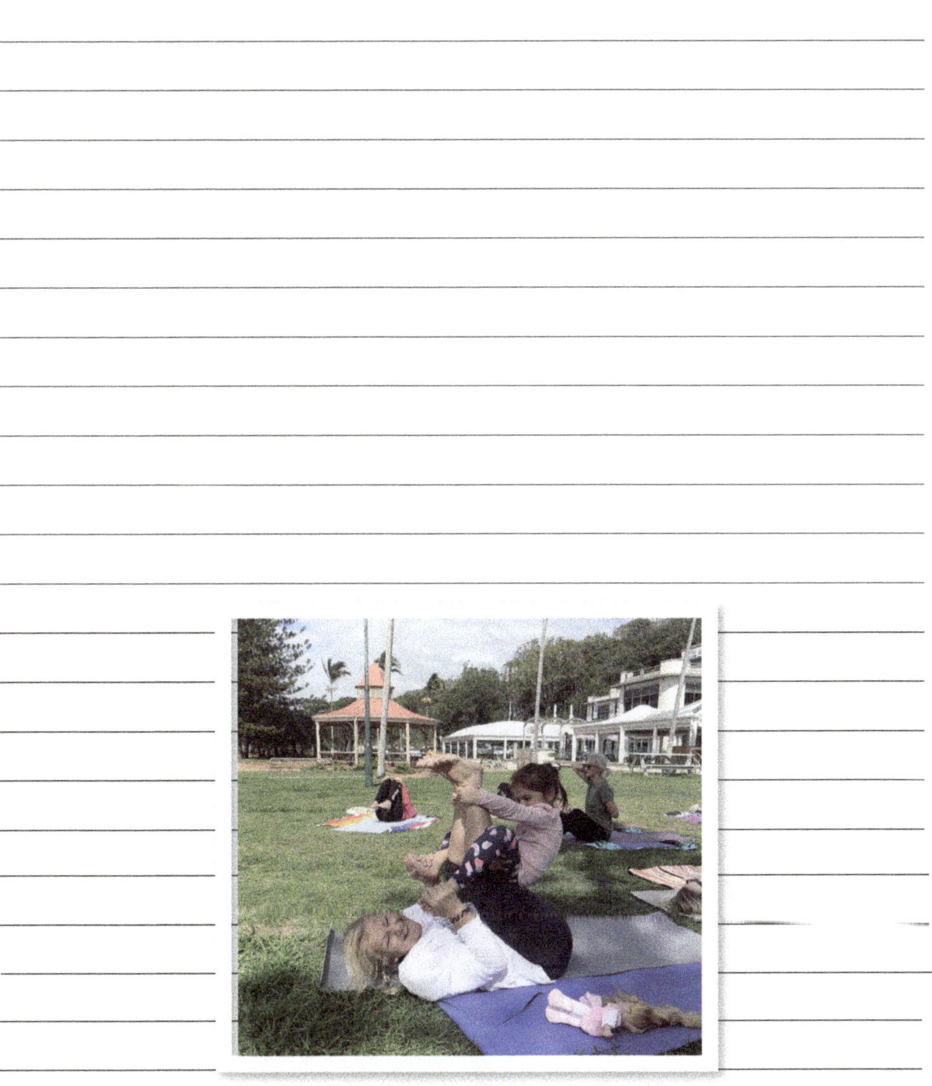

positive AFFIRMATION

I grow stronger by choice

acceptance

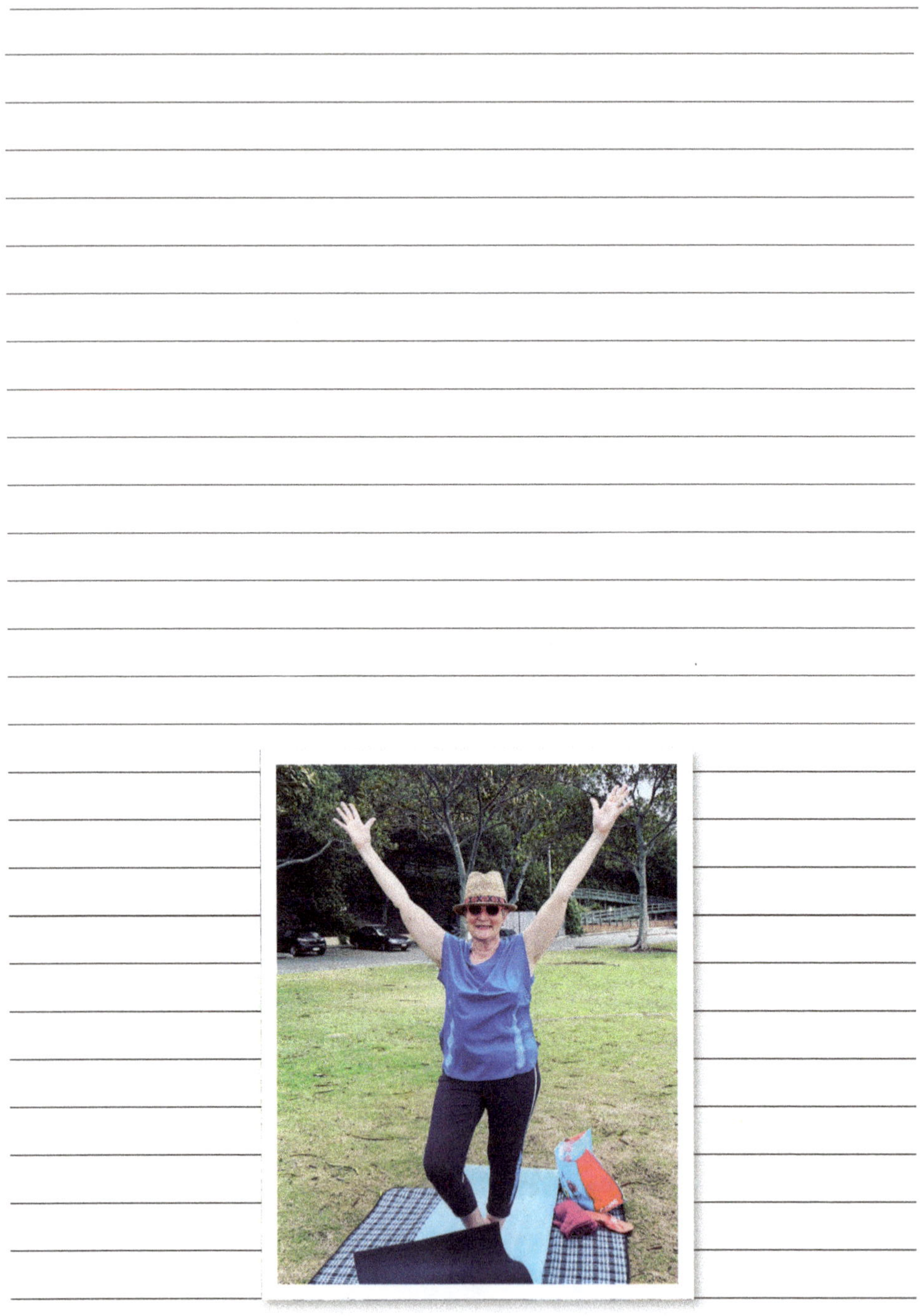

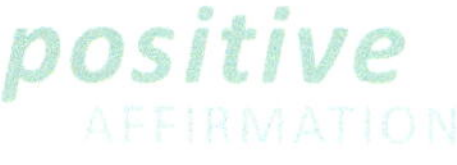

I choose joy

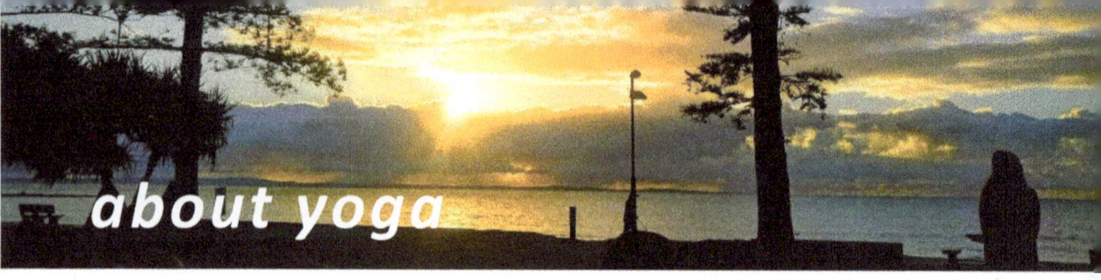

Connecting mind and body into a spiritual union

Yoga began thousands of years ago and is now embraced by Western culture for its ability to strengthen, stretch and tone the body whilst calming and relaxing the mind.

Yoga improves immunity, digestion, and increases happy hormones. It lowers blood pressure, decreases body fat, and strengthens lean muscle tissue. With yoga you will regain the agility and flexibility you thought was only possible in your youth.

Yoga can be practised at any age. Many yogis in their eighties and nineties still balance and stretch as they did fifty years earlier. Recent studies have shown that elderly people who practise yoga maintain active brain tissue, and have fewer falls.

Breathing

The deep breathing practised in yoga decreases anxiety, improves circulation, raises immunity, facilitates healing and promotes energy.

Throughout yoga, breathe deeply into postures, relaxing muscles as you exhale. For a simple guide to breathing, breathe in for five-eight seconds and out for six-nine seconds. There are many types of breath practised through yoga, and this simple breath will guide you towards the first step in regaining your health and vitality.

Mindfulness

The mindfulness of yoga encourages you to accept life here and now. As you move into postures you will notice your inner talk. If you are critical towards yourself, this shows how you treat yourself in life. Breathe deeply and let go of judgement. Use affirmations like, "I love and accept myself, just as I am." Doing this in yoga will help you
love and accept yourself in daily life.

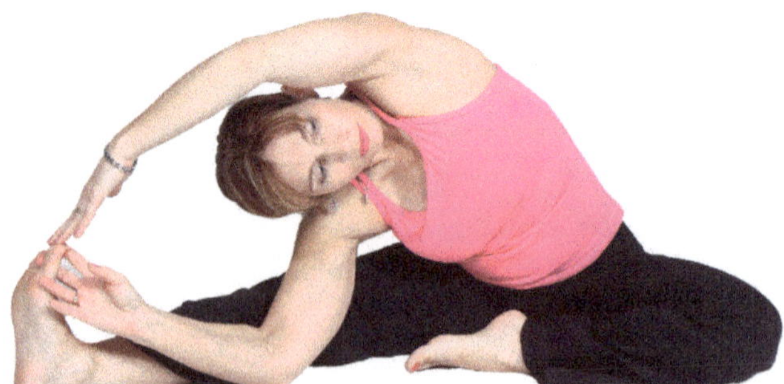

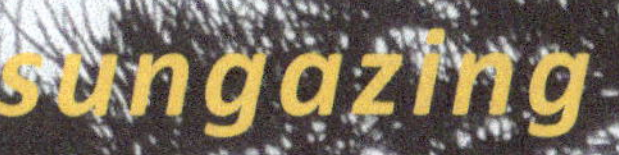

In winter we catch the sunrise during our yoga class.
We stop whatever we are doing and spend one minute sun gazing.

Sungazing activates your pineal gland.
It sets your body clock and increases happy and calm hormones.

How to Sungaze

Face the sunrise. Gaze somewhere along the horizon, allowing the full spectrum of light to enter your eyes and activate your pineal gland (remember to take off your sunnies).

Breathe deeply

Your pineal gland sits in the centre of your brain and is about the size of a grape. Imagine your pineal gland is like a tiny golden sun, filled with pure positive energy.
As you sun gaze, it is shining its rays to your entire endocrine system.
Your pineal gland will boost happy hormones, your immune system, and switch on your body clock.
Spend the next minute breathing deeply as the sun rises...
You are already perfect...
You are already beautiful...

You are already whole...

Love...

Peace...

Joy...

Deep breath in...and release..*Well done.*

SUN SALUTATIONS

Honour your body, go at your own pace, breathe deeply

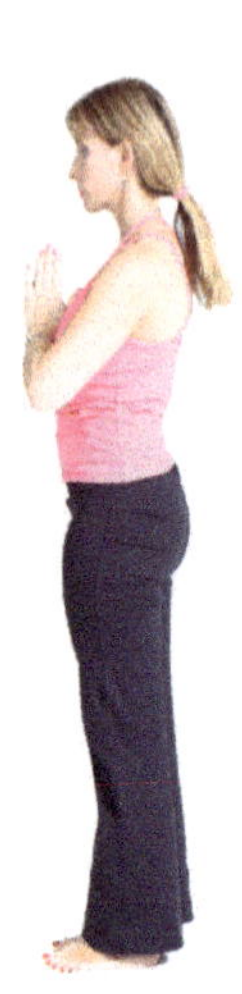

1. Hands to heart

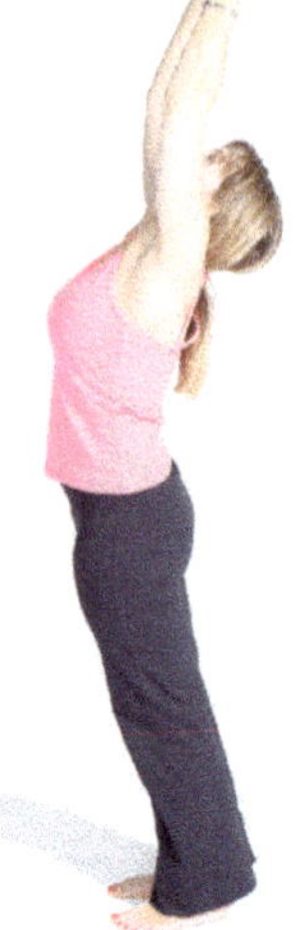

2. Breathe in, *reach back*

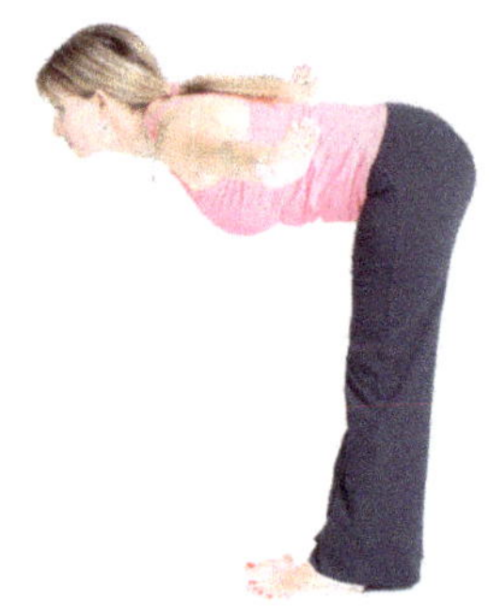

3. Breathe out, *Swan Dive* into *Forward Fold*

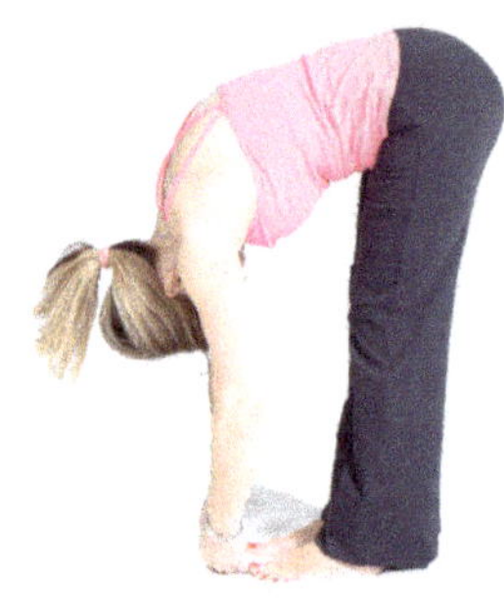

4. Pause and breath

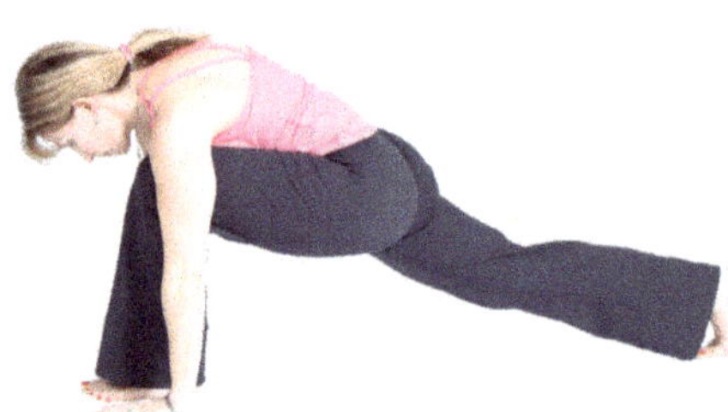

5. Place hands and step right foot back for a *Lunge*

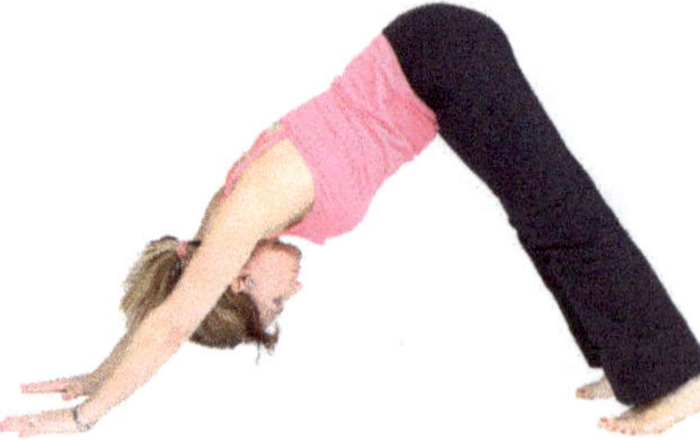

6. From *Lunge* step into *Downward Facing Dog*

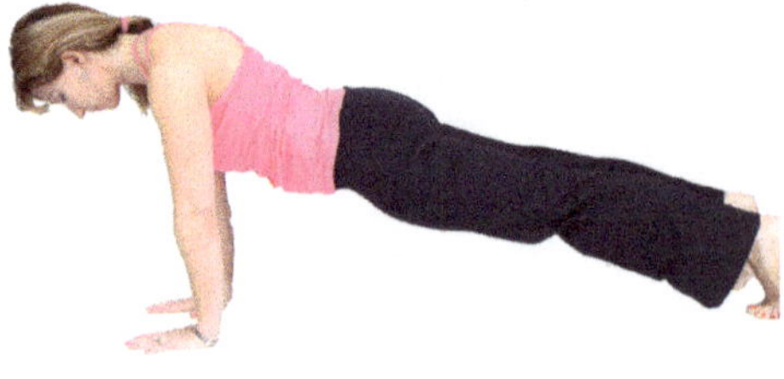

7. From *Downwad Dog* Breathe in to *Plank* and pause for one breath

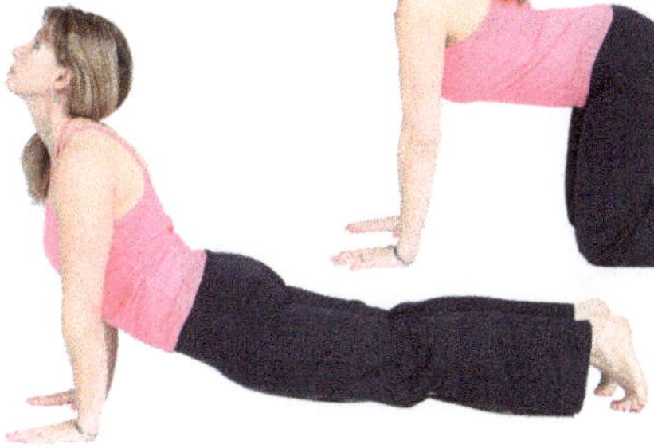

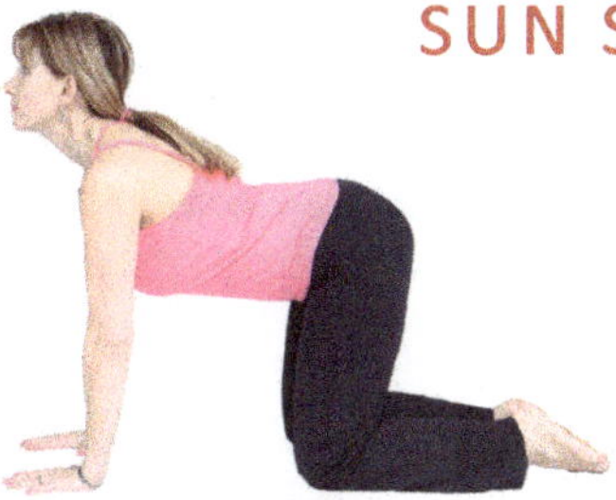

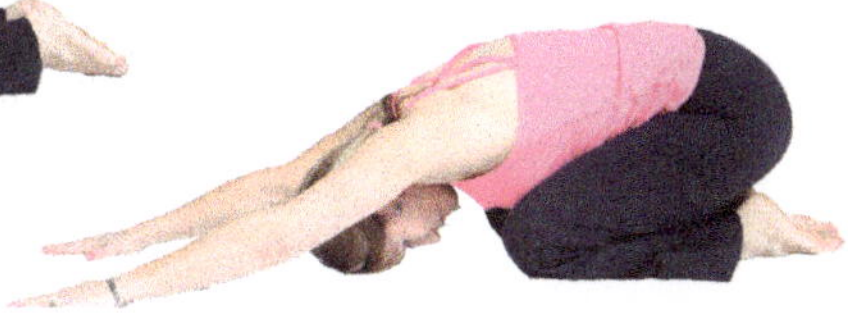

8. From *Plank*, place knees to earth for *Cow pose* for option one, or *Upward* Facing *Dog* for option two

09. Breathe out to *Swan pose.* *Pause for one breath*

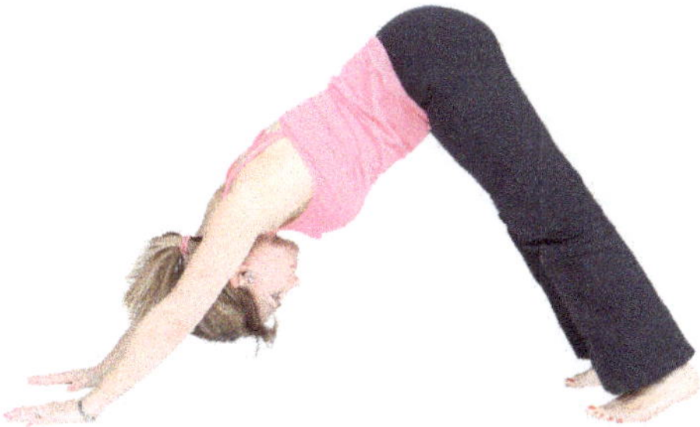

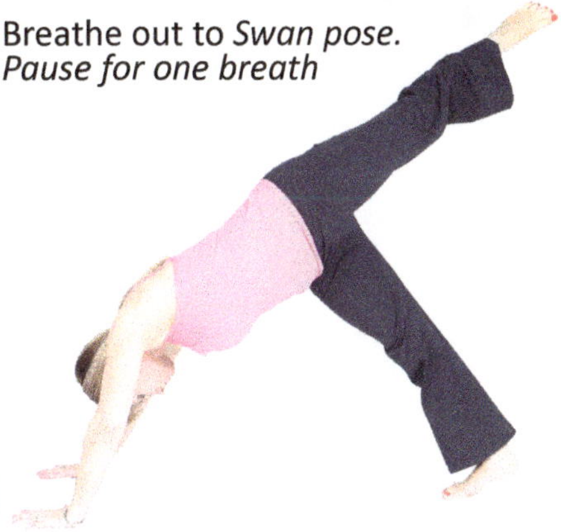

10. From *Swan pose*, breathe and lift into *Downward Dog.* Then lift right leg up for *Three Legged Dog.* Scoop leg through to *Lunge*

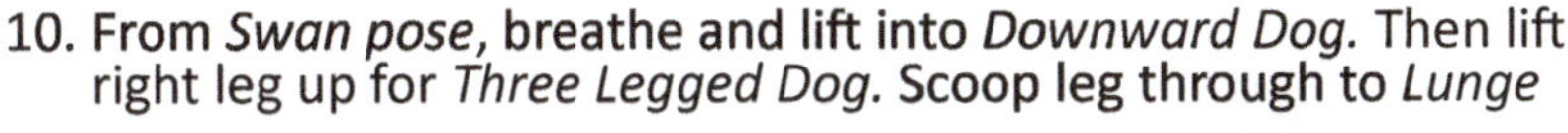

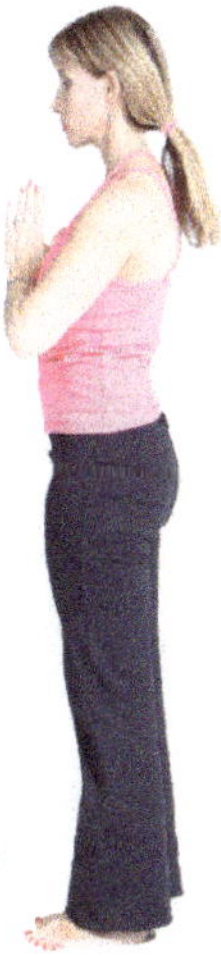

11. From *Lunge* bring the back leg forward into *Forward Fold*

12. From *Forward Fold*, breathe and softly rise, bring hands back to heart. *Repeat with left leg*

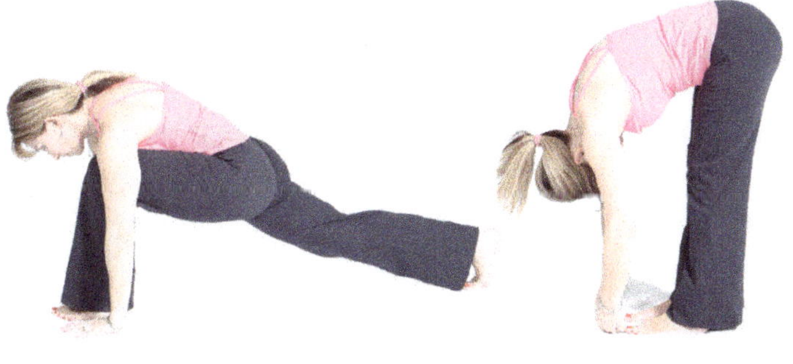

Practise this sequence as many times as your body needs

life is like yoga

Yoga reflects life. Some days are easy, some days are hard.

The more you accept yourself in each posture, the easier it is to deepen and move forward. The more you can accept 'you are where you are' in life, the easier it becomes to move forward.

Acceptance

Acceptance is important because it lets go of tension and resistance. When it is difficult to accept life's changes, your body sets up resistance. This resistance eventually becomes tension, and if left unresolved, can create dis-ease in the body. Acceptance is easier than approval. You may not like what is happening, but you can accept it is happening. As soon as acceptance is allowed, tension resolves, and life softens.

Expect good things

When you allow yourself to relax into the moment, wonderful things happen. The resistance leaves and positive options move in. When you let go of worry, solutions appear. When you let go of trying so hard, synchronicity occurs.

The brain grows and connects neurons every time you have a thought or experience. If you train yourself to find the best in a situation (even if it's imaginary), positive expectation grows. And the brain will look for, and find, more positive outcomes.

When you believe something, you reflect that belief through your actions and thoughts. This can have negative consequences (like the person who believes they can't achieve) or it can have positive consequences (like the person who believes they can do great things). You can change a negative pattern into a positive pattern by using focus.

Train yourself to look for things you like rather than things you don't like. The more you find things you like, the more you will attract experiences that bring you joy.

Focus on what you want

In all situations, there is a choice on what to focus on. If you make a conscious effort to look for things you like, you will be training your mind towards what is wanted, rather than what is unwanted.

You can do this. You are already doing this.
Give yourself a break and realise how wonderful you really are.

I was on my yoga mat looking at the blue sky, clouds and trees, when I noticed a plastic bag stuck in a tree. I stared at it for ages.

'What's that doing there?' I wondered. I started thinking about rubbish and how fast food affects us - and before I knew it, I had shifted myself away from feeling positive (trees grass beach clouds sky friends peace calm) and I was focusing on the tiniest piece gone wrong (one bag in the tree).

I knew that if I kept looking at that bag for long enough, I would forget the peace around me, and start noticing the bits of rubbish on the ground, and that person over there smoking, and the noise from the passing truck, and the ache in my back.

Am I controlling what I focus on? I wondered. Do I really have the ability to feel good or feel bad? Maybe I do. I took my eyes away from the rubbish and started looking at the trees again. I stayed focused. Soon I noticed another shift; a deeper breath and stillness.

It is so easy, yet I have to remind myself to do it. I have decided that today I will commit to looking for what is right in my world. I will talk about what is working. I will focus on the good that is already here, and see what happens. We deserve that, right?

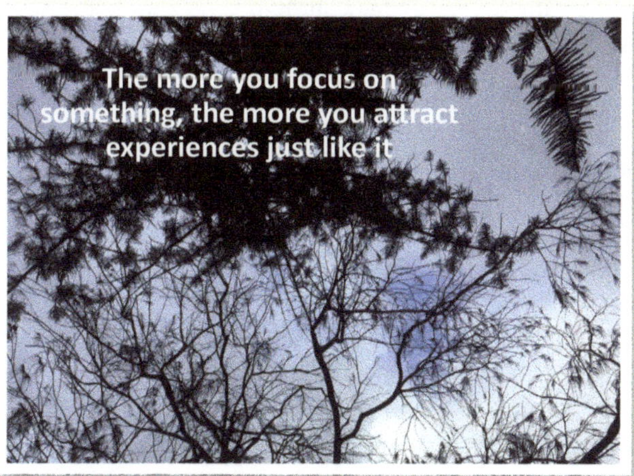

Your Yoga Practise

Create a space where you can move freely, breathe deeply and play ambient music.

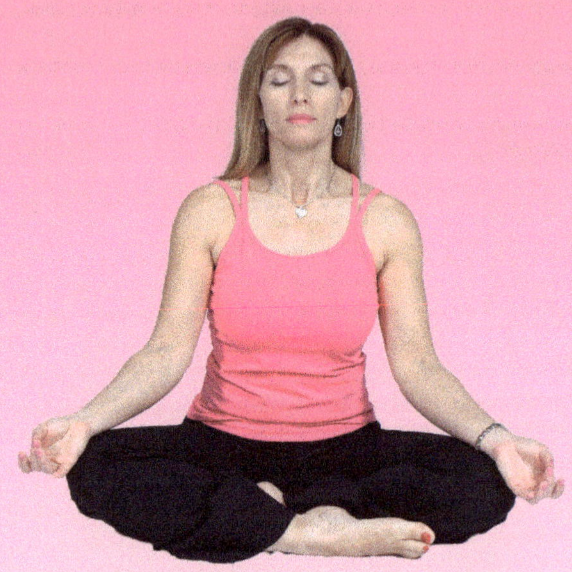

CIRCLE OF JOY

Peace

Begin in a mindful meditation to help clear your mind and relax your body.

Sit in a comfortable position. You can lay your hands on your knees with palms open to the sky to increase your connection to the universe, or palms down for grounding.

Close your eyes. Lengthen the spine, relax shoulders, close eyes and take deep breaths until you feel peaceful and relaxed.. Bring your awareness to your third eye (the space between your eyebrows). Breathe into your abdomen and feel your lungs expand with each breath. If you feel any tension in your body, breathe into the tension and let it go.

Set your intention for today's yoga practice. You may want to increase strength, peace, flexibility, balance or clarity. Reflect as you breathe in and out. Breathe in and out through the nose. Breathe in peace and breathe out tension. Find the centre of your heart.

Breathe in a slow and steady rhythm,
pause at the beginning and end of each breath.

Bring hands to heart: inhale,
interlace fingers and lift hands
under chin.

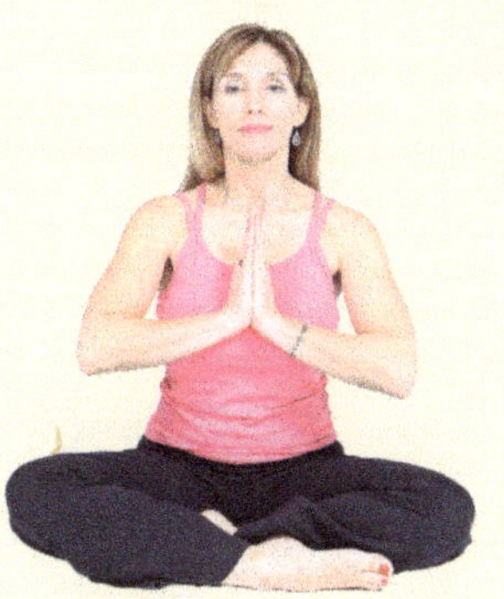

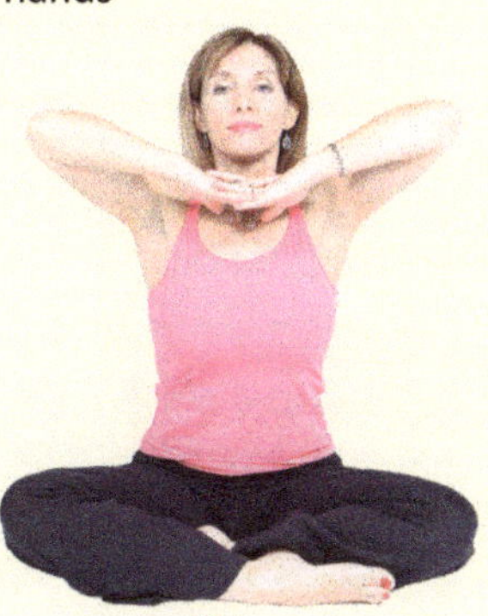

Exhale, press hands forward,
press back away. Inhale,
stretch arms up.

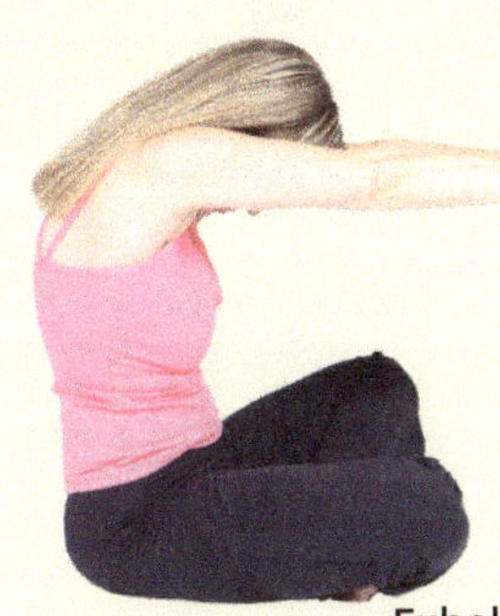

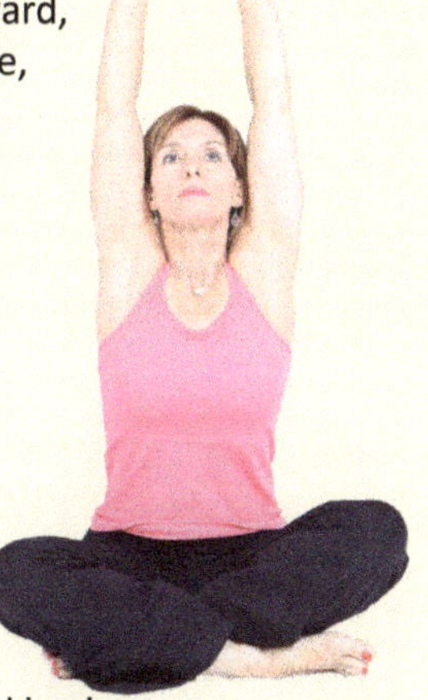

Exhale bring hands behind back
and clasp hands. Inhale, bring
hands back to heart. Repeat.

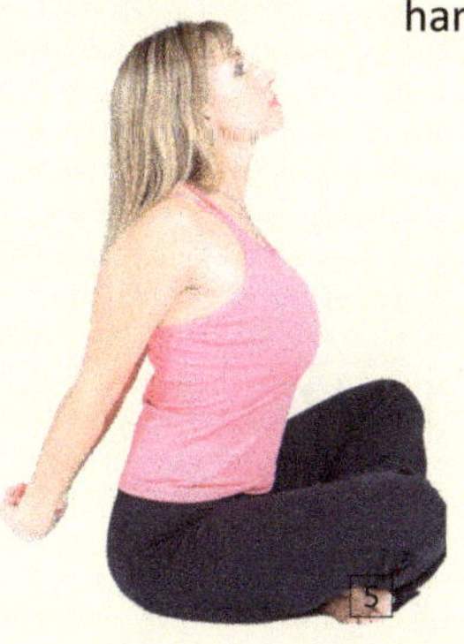

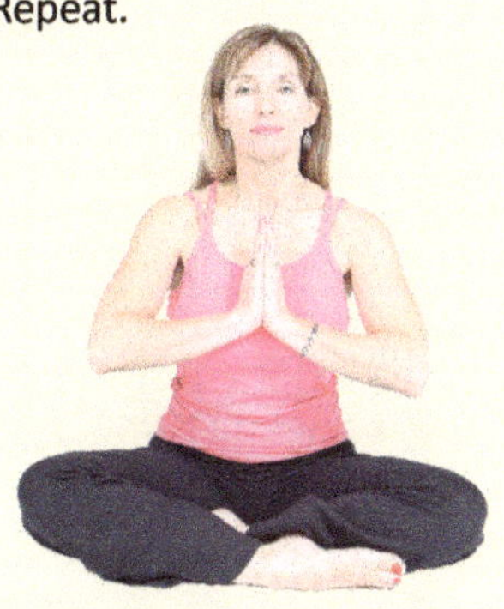

SIDE BEND

Bring hands to heart. Inhale and stretch both arms up and reach one hand to the side as the other reaches over.

Relax shoulders and press hips towards the floor. Rotate back shoulder forward and open heart.

Hold the pose for a few breaths, and change sides. Finish by crossing right arm over left knee for Seated Spinal Twist.

Relax your heart and let love in

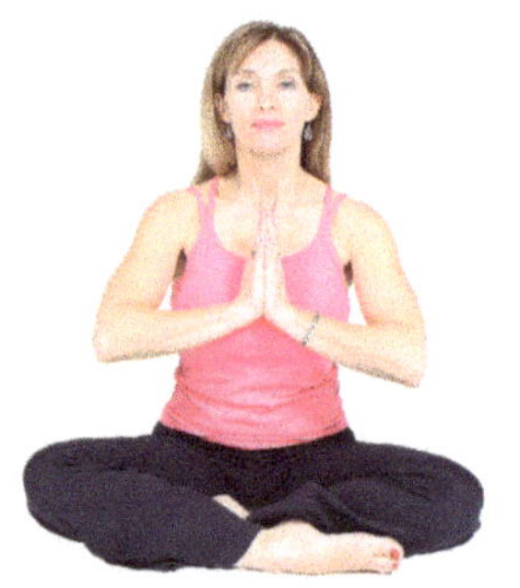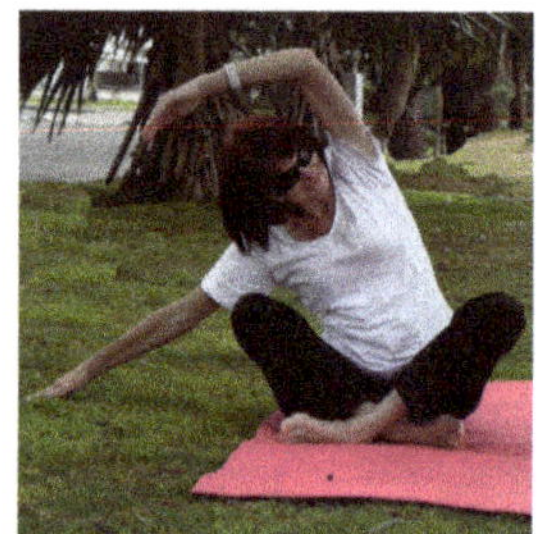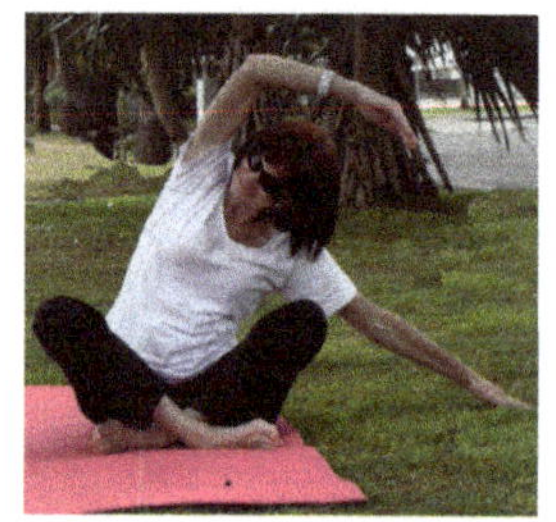

SEATED SPINAL TWIST

Releases spine tension, increases circulation to organs.

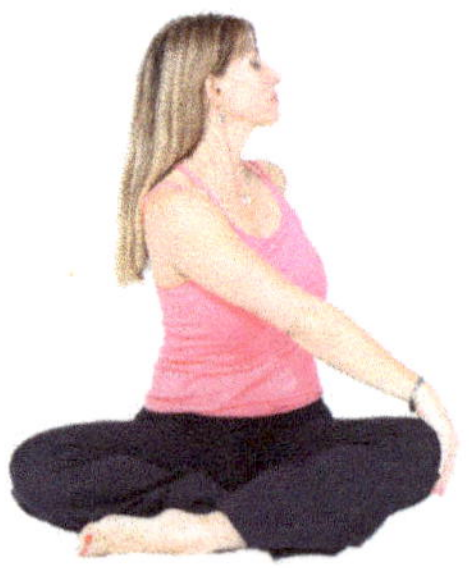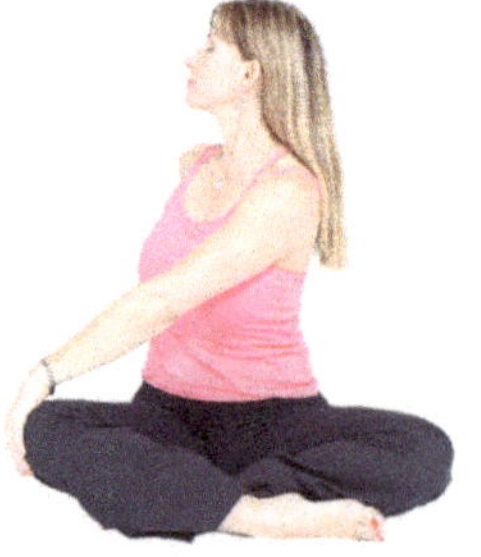

In a cross-legged or half lotus, cross right arm over left knee and place left hand near tailbone.

Inhale to lengthen the spine, exhale to twist. Press towards the back. Stay for three or four breaths, releasing to the front on exhale.

Change sides.

Love yourself for who you are in this moment

SEATED
FORWARD FOLD

Relax spine

Interlace fingers, inhale
reach up to the sky and reach back.

Exhale, press forward,
tuck tailbone down,
fold arms onto the floor
and rest head.

Stay for several deep breaths.

Breathe deeply

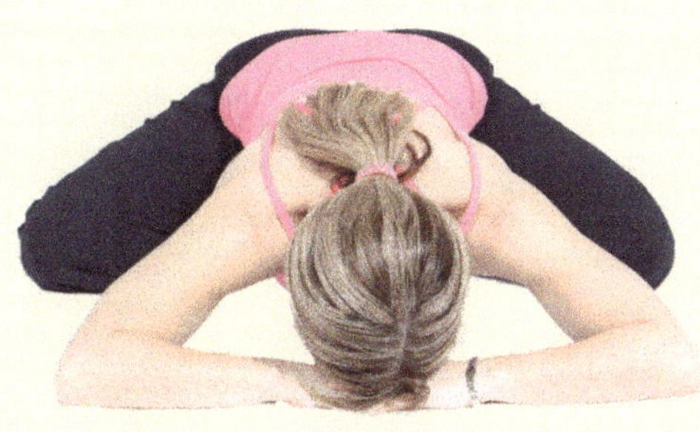

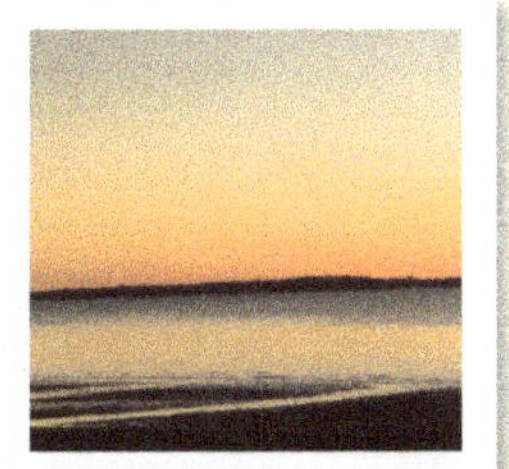
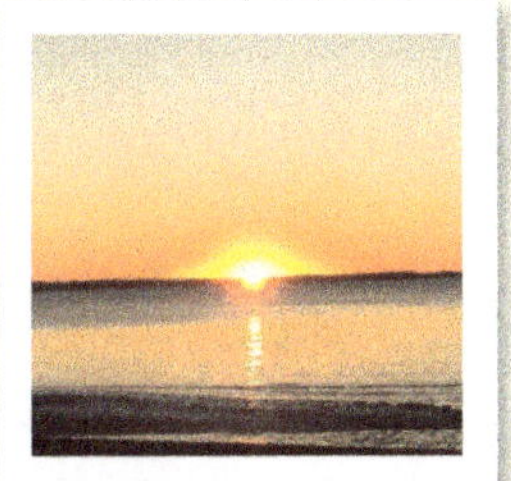
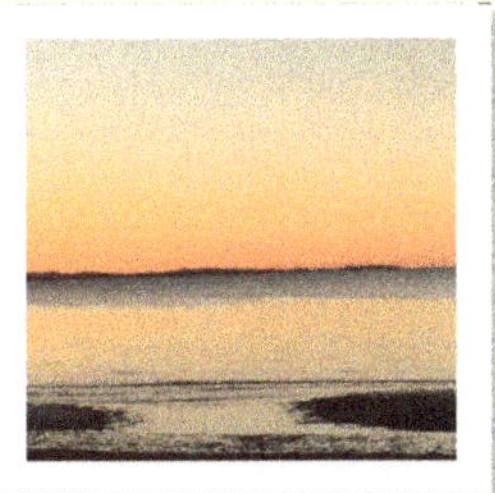

peace

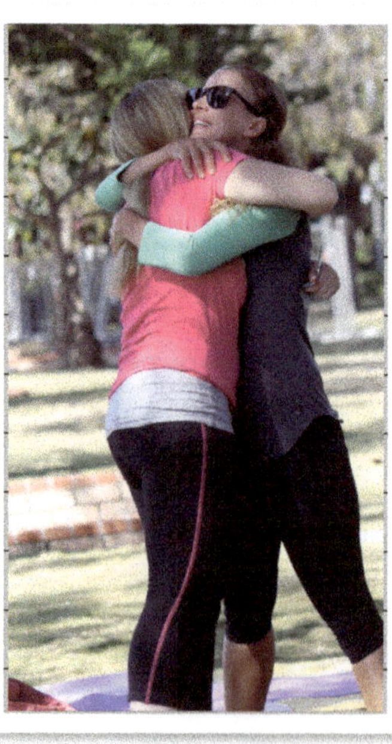

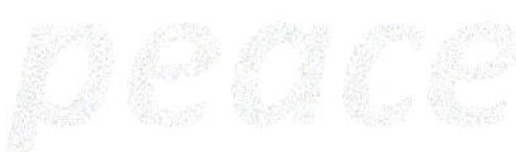

positive
AFFIRMATION

I love, honour and accept myself in this moment

love

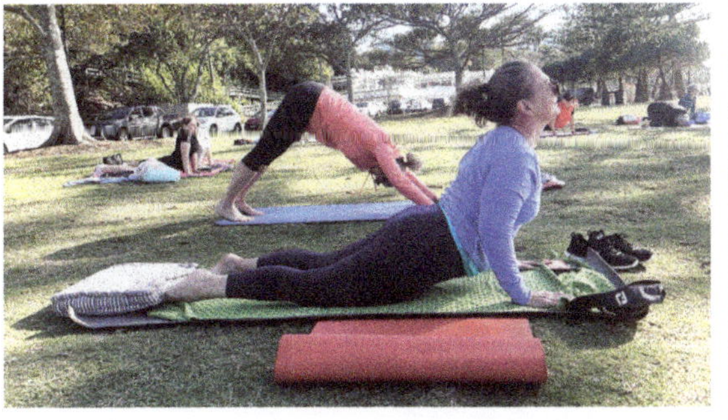

positive
AFFIRMATION

I invite joy and fun into my life

joy

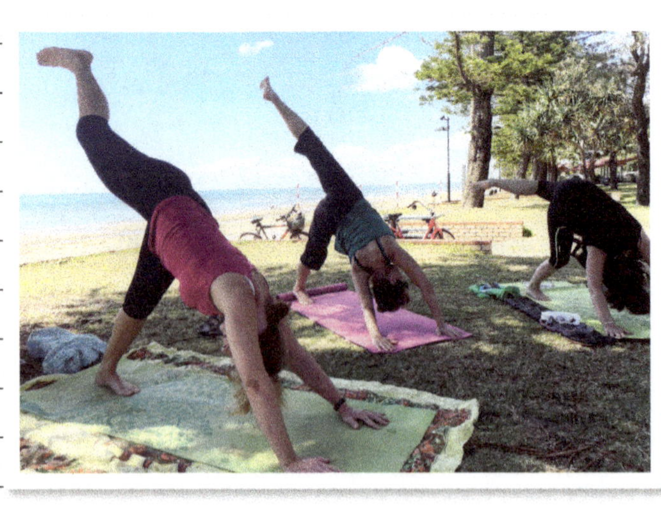

Connection is key

happiness

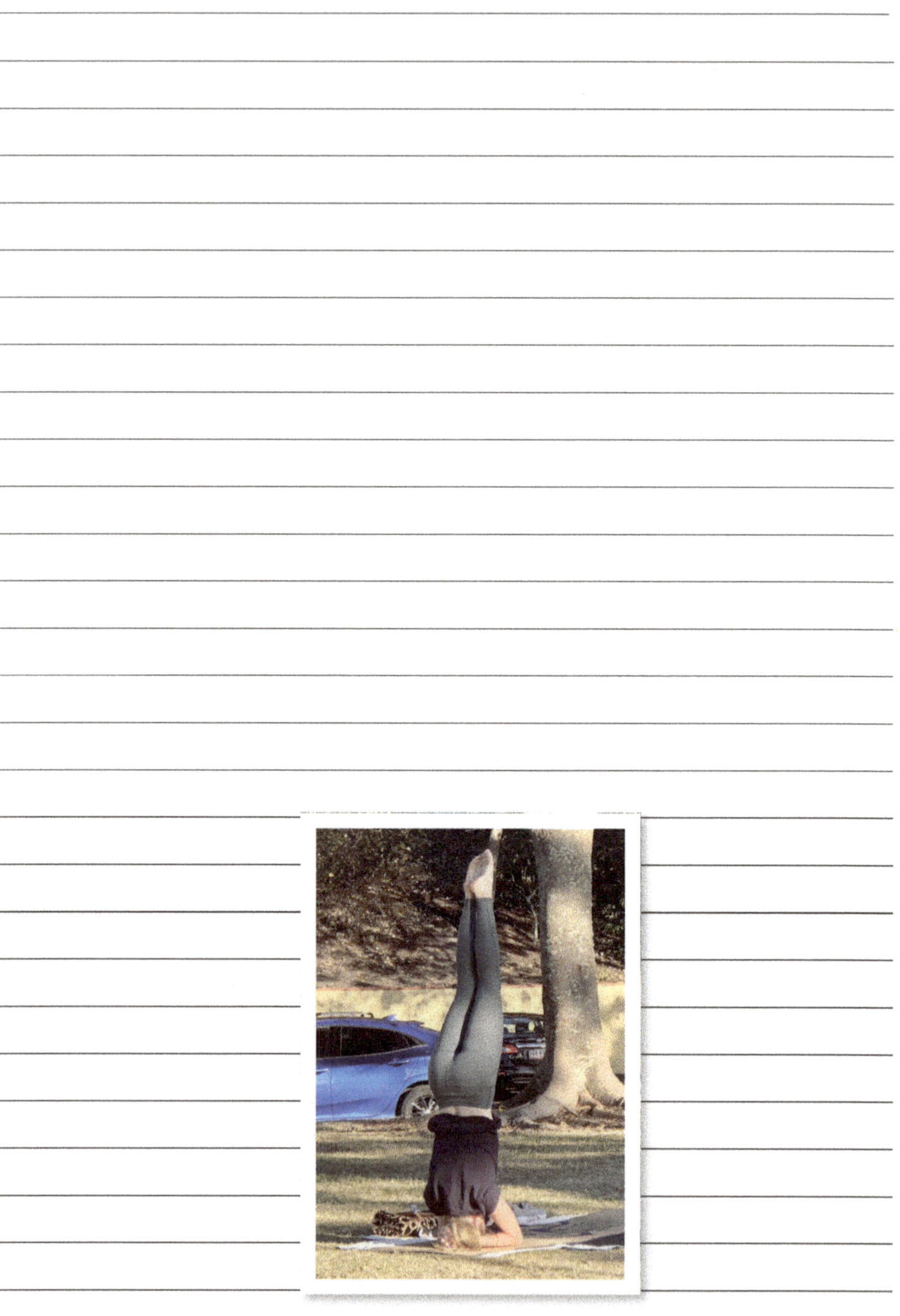

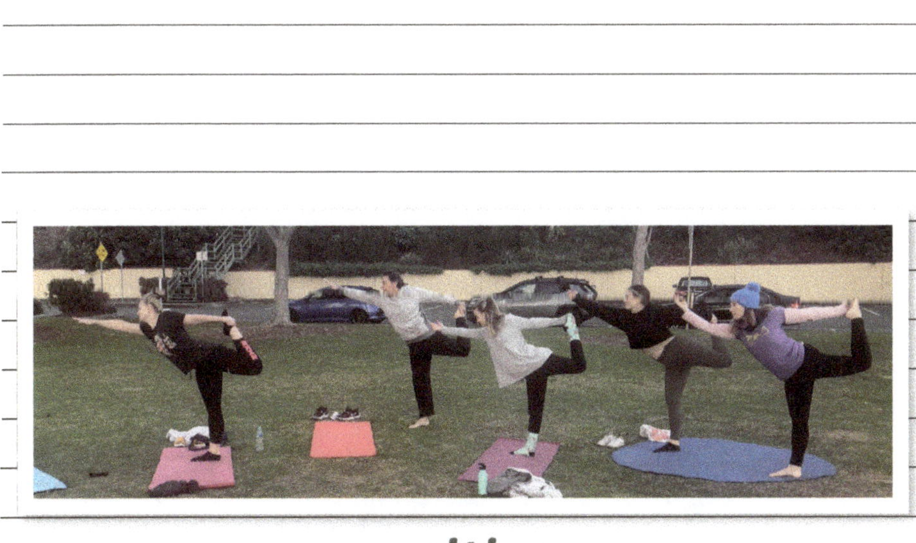

positive
AFFIRMATION

Expect good things and look forward to your life

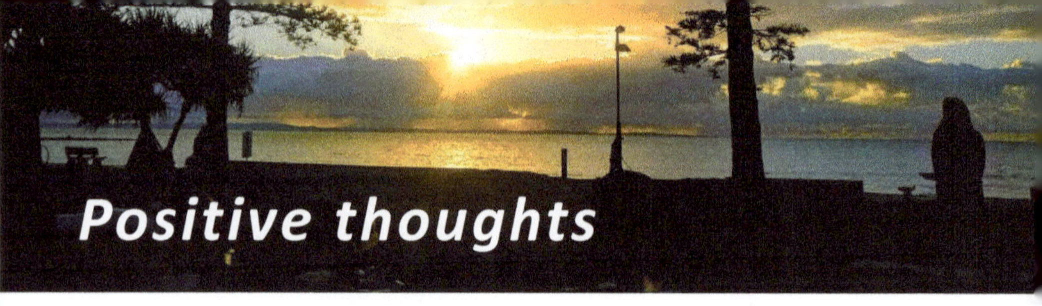

Positive thoughts

There is positive and negative in every situation. By focusing on the positive, you train your mind to positive habits, which will help you attract more positive experiences.

This means you will be healthier and happier, just by looking for things you like, rather than things you don't like. It's easy to find things you like when things are going your way, but what about when they're not?

If you find yourself in a negative thought pattern, no matter what it is or why you are experiencing it, take a few moments to look for things you like. By focusing on something positive you will create a shift in how you are feeling and what you are attracting.

It doesn't matter how small the thought starts. When I first decided to change my life, I was working in a job that didn't allow me to grow. I started pretending I was empowered and in charge. That I loved my job. I started to focus on things (real and imagined) that bought me joy.

Even though I was suffering from depression and would continue to do so for a number of years, I persisted.

After a few months of retraining my focus, I started thinking about a yoga class on the beach. The more I thought about it, the more I liked the idea. I quit my job (that took time and courage), invited my friends to join me, and drove to the beach for my first class. One person showed up, but that was okay, because I was happy to be doing what I loved.

For the first 7 months there were a regular two to four people coming to class. As my marketing and confidence improved, more people came. Friends started bringing friends, and I began meeting people who were aligned with myself.

After one year, 10 to 20 people came regularly and our yoga family was formed.

You don't need to be happy all the time to attract
a better life, you just need to keep leaning towards
a better feeling and a better thought for better
experiences to come to you.

We have been doing yoga on the beach for more than eleven years now, and we hold 5 - 7 classes a week. Our classes and our social calander is full. We embrace every new person that comes to class, and our class has expanded to include children that come for free, and dogs that come to play.

In 2011 we published our first yoga book and had a cocktail launch. In 2014 we published *Yoga for Little Bears* with some great work from graphic designers Jane Watt and Jamie Palmer, and editors Narelle Douglass and Jane Todd. Every year since, Monica has published eBooks and sells online to teachers and parents.

In 2018 we created a documentary on 'Yoga in Redcliffe' with filmmaker Graeme Collins. In 2019 we featured on the BBC show *'Wanted Down Under.'*

In 2020 we faced our biggest challenge - the lockdown. In a matter of weeks our classes and social life and freedom were taken away. Many of our friends were self-isolating and our dreams were shattered. Monica took this opportunity to take her yoga classes onto facebook live so everyone could join in. It gave us the chance to spend time together, chat on video and stay centred and strong to weather this time.

We embrace the yoga philosophy of living life as fully and as lovingly as we can. Each class focuses on lifting our vibrations to it's highest potential so that we can continue to attract health, peace, freedom and prosperity for us all.

Creating a balanced and purposeful life is a life-long journey, but the moment you begin your world starts to change. In time, you will look back and say, 'Look how far I've come'.

One small shift can change your world.

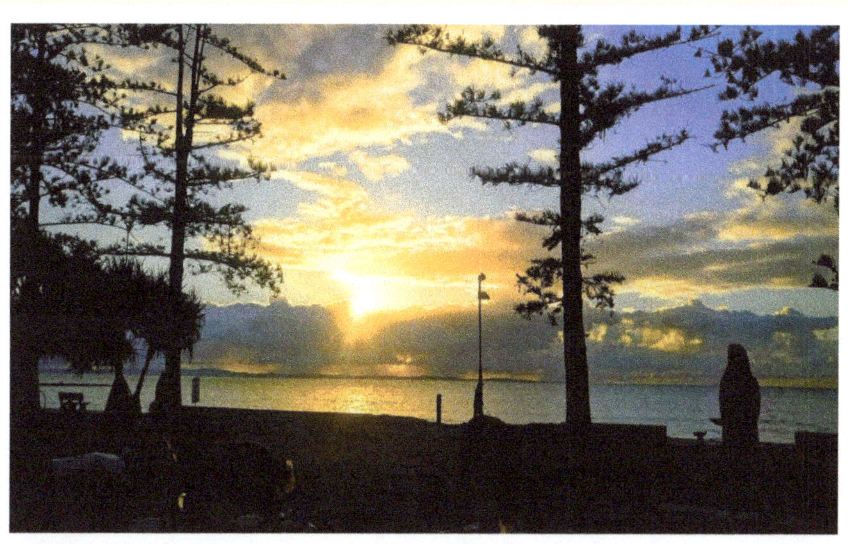

Release and Repair

Place hands beneath shoulders and knees beneath hips. Do *Cat-Cow pose* when your back is tense, and to warm up for stronger poses such as *Arm-Leg extension* and *Up-Dog-Down-Dog*.

CAT - COW

Full breath out for *Cat* as you press hands into the earth, lengthen arms, tuck tailbone under and lift *pelvic floor.* Full breath in to *Cow* as you lift tailbone, arch the spine and lift head. Repeat for a few minutes.

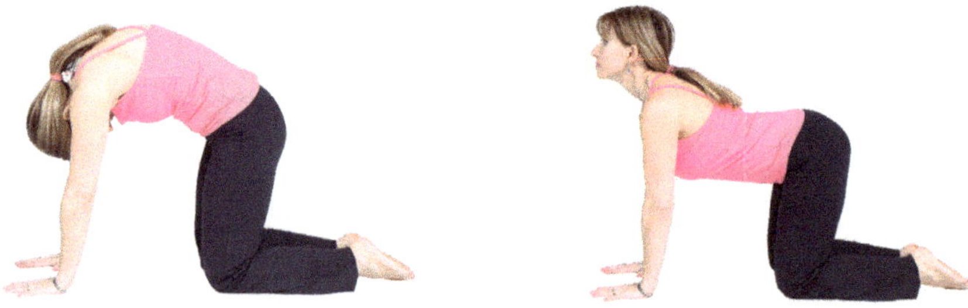

UP-DOG - SWAN

Up Dog; place hands beneath shoulders and knees beneath hips. Press hips forward, tuck the arms towards ribs, lift heart and press in pelvic floor. Swan pose, press back towards heels. Outstretch arms.

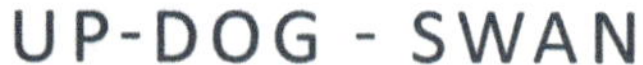

UP-DOG - SWAN

From *Up-Dog*, place heels towards earth, and press into the *Down-Dog*. In *Down Dog*, press heart towards thighs, lift tailbone towards the sky,
relax the head.

ARM AND LEG EXTENSION

*Strengthens and lengthens lower back,
spine and hamstrings*

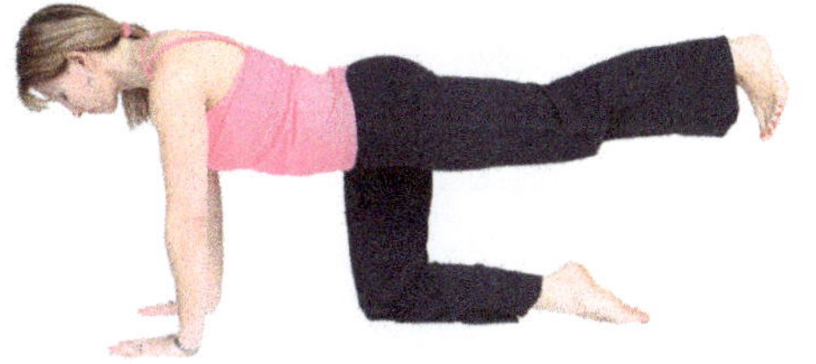

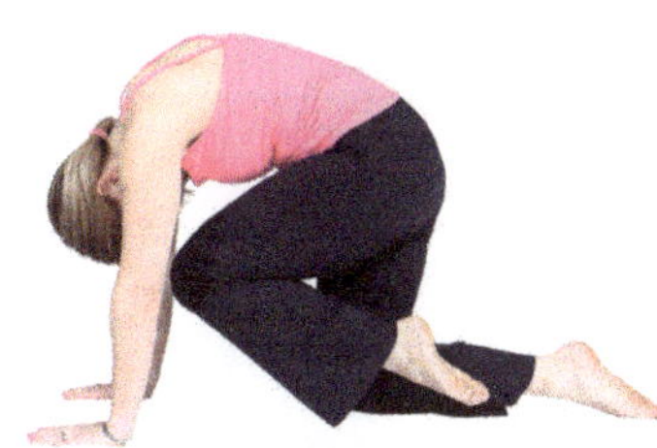

Inhale to extend leg behind. Keep
hips parallel with the floor,
lift pelvic floor.

Exhale and fold knee
towards head. For a
stronger option, add the
opposite arm in extension
and place hand to knee.

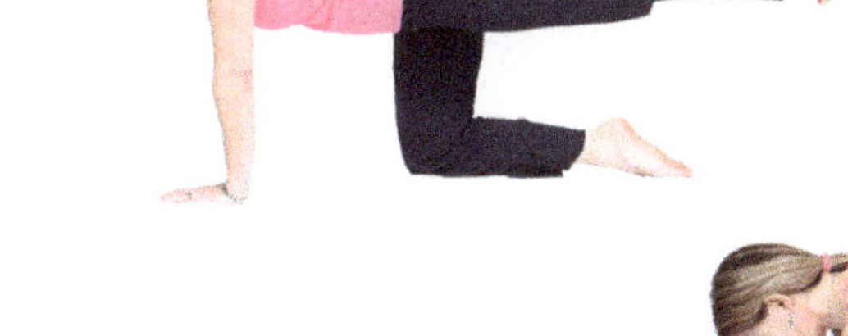

Repeat ten times holding the last
repetition for ten seconds. Stay in
extension for option one, move into
Half-Bow for option two.

WIDE-LEGGED CHILD

Releases groin and inner thighs

Open knees, keep big toes together,
inhale and press buttocks to heels
and release body to the earth.

Relax for one minute before repeating
Release and Repair, and *Arm-Leg extension*
for the other side.

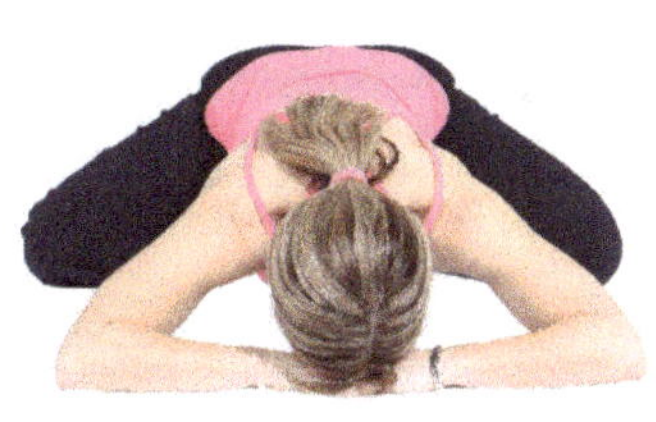

YOGA kids

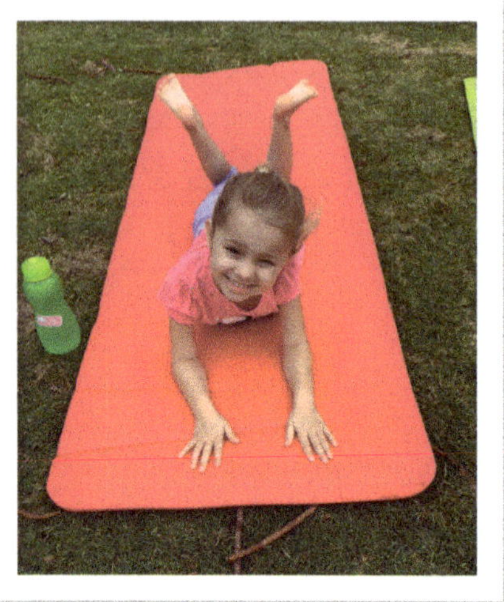

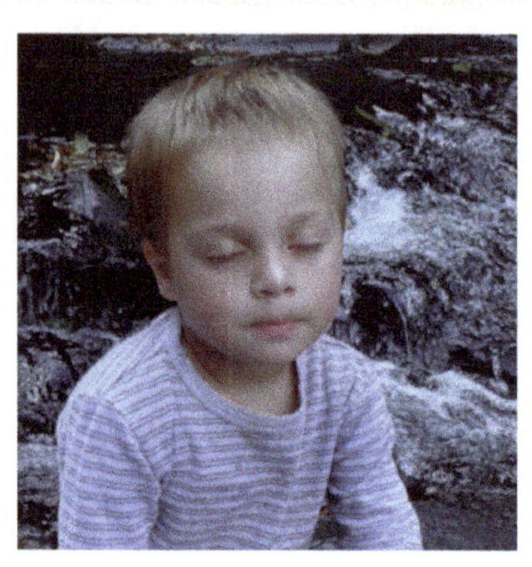

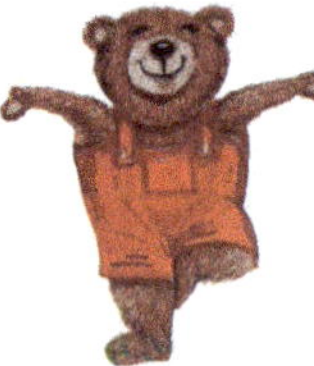

YOGA bear

YOGA parents

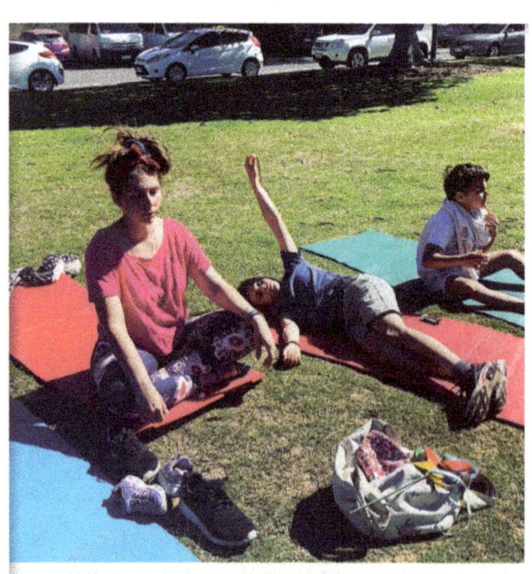

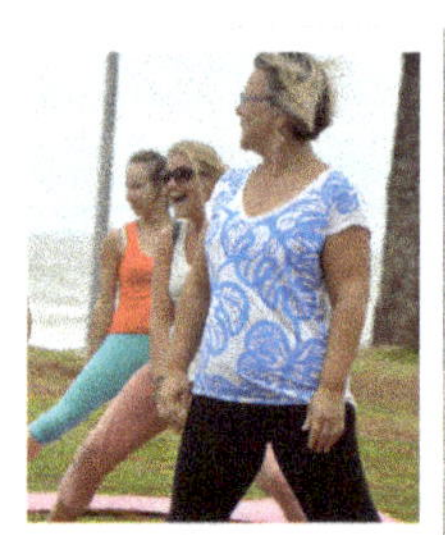

YOUNG 50s

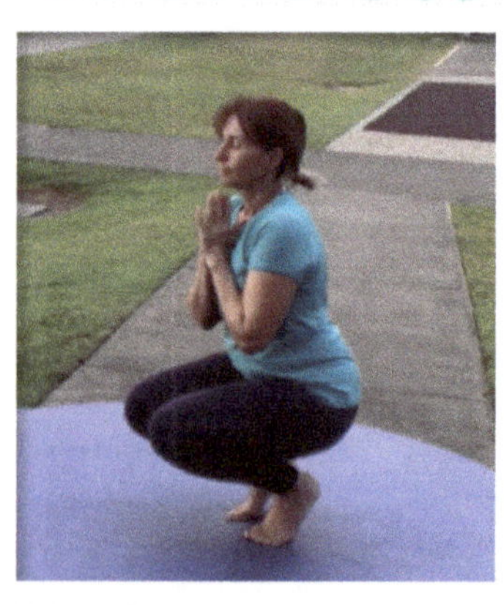

FIT 60s

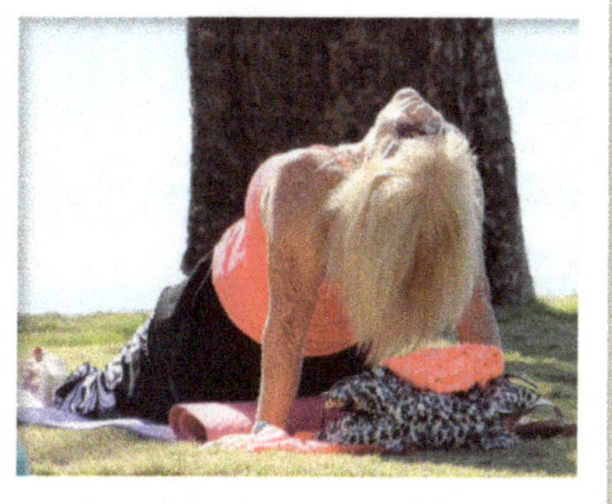

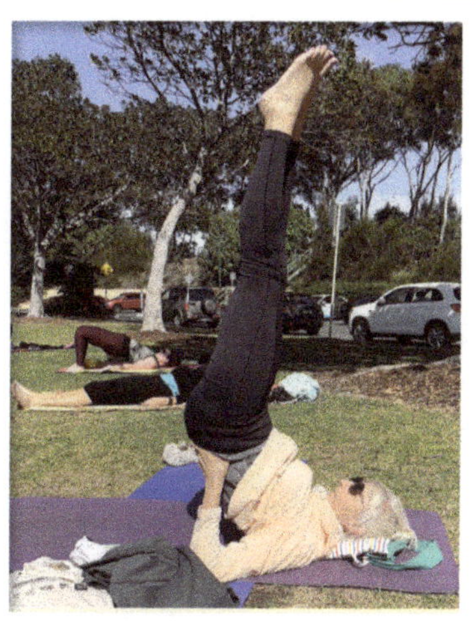

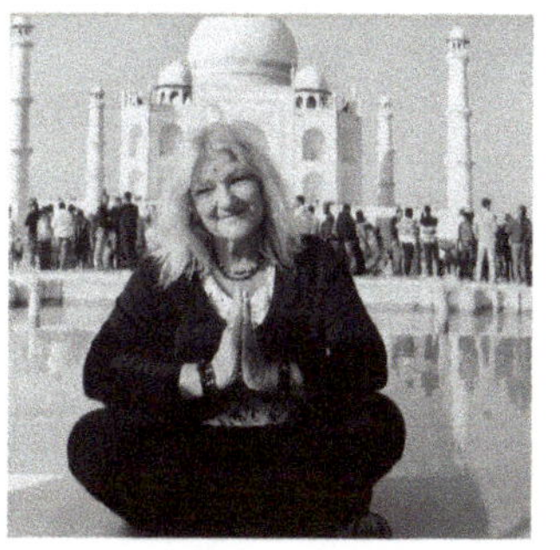

AWESOME 70s

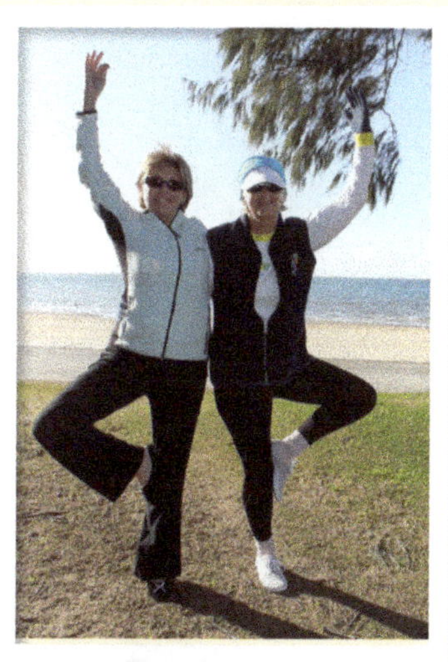

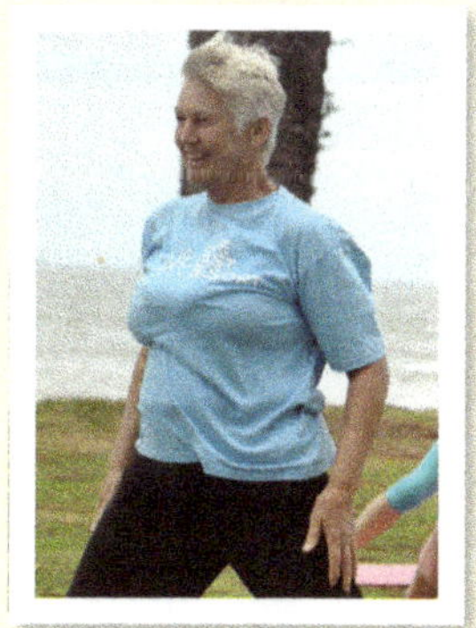

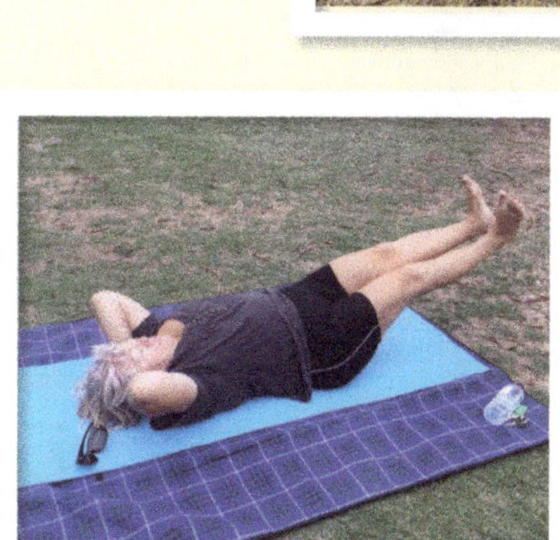

YOGA
LOVE

self-care

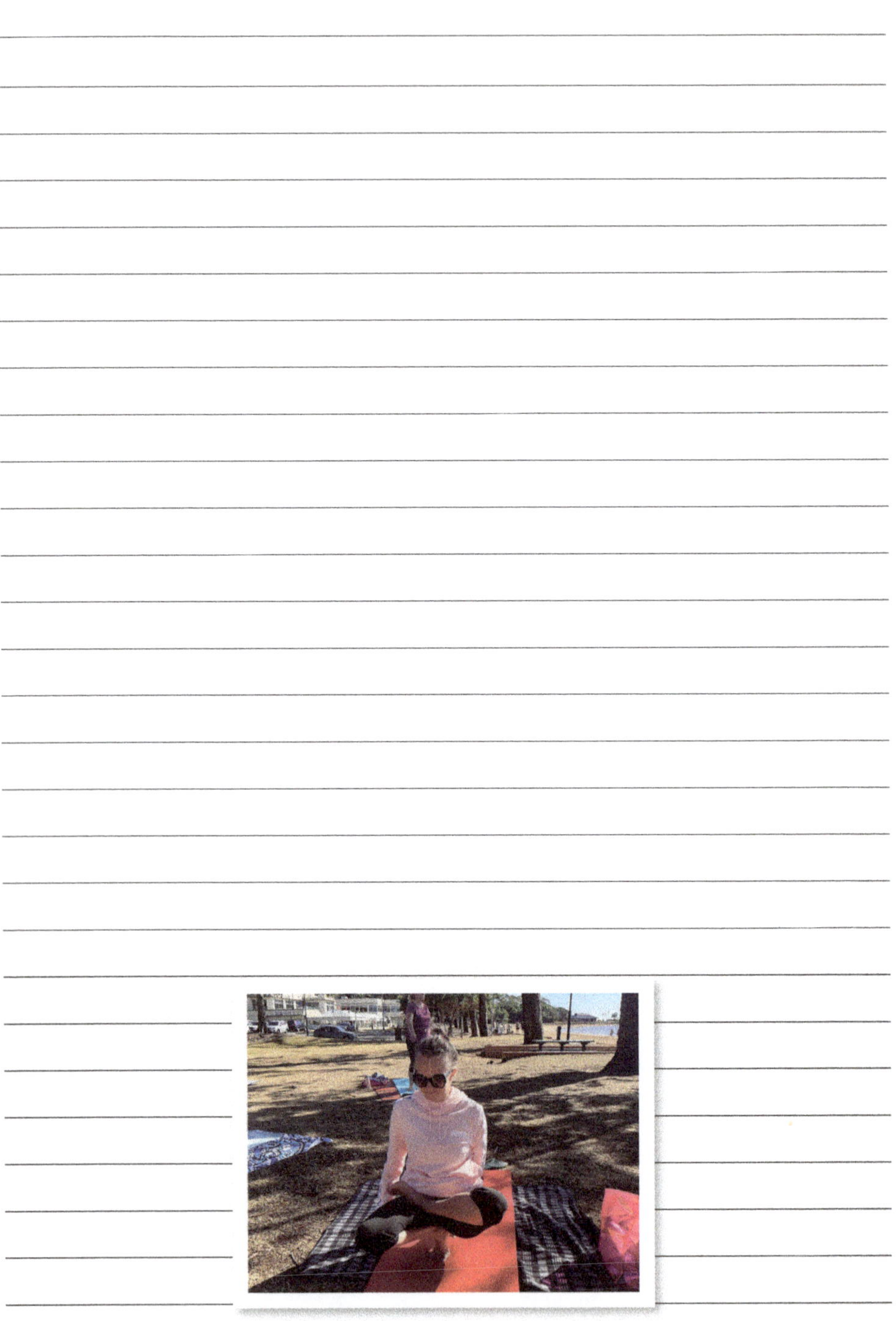

positive
AFFIRMATION

I am the hero I was hoping to find

self-esteem

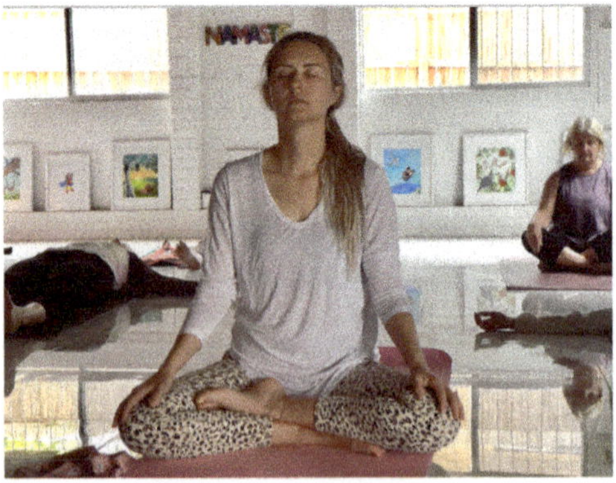

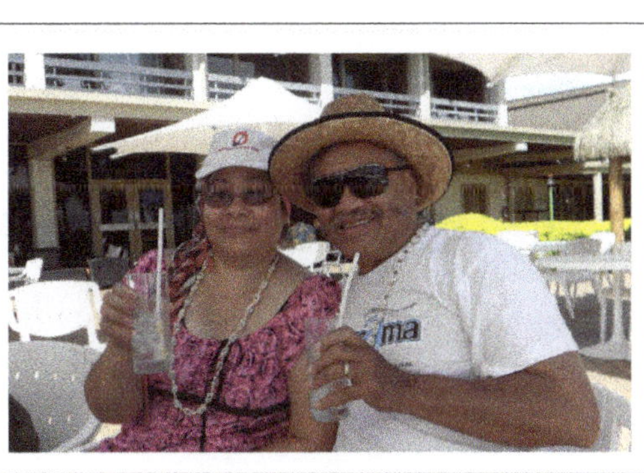

positive
AFFIRMATION

I believe in myself and I follow my dreams

enthusiasm

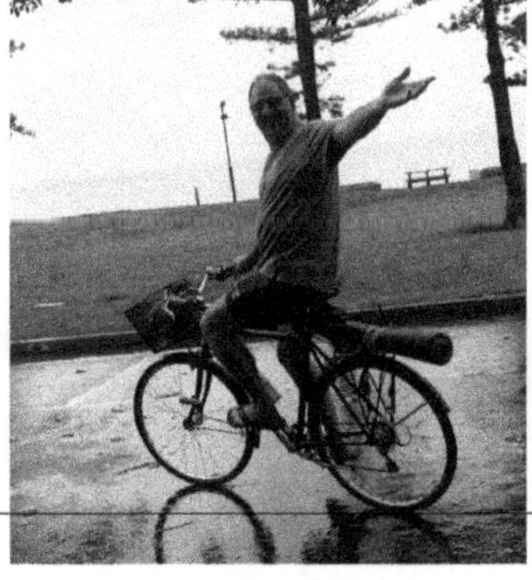

positive
AFFIRMATION

I believe in myself and I follow my heart

generosity

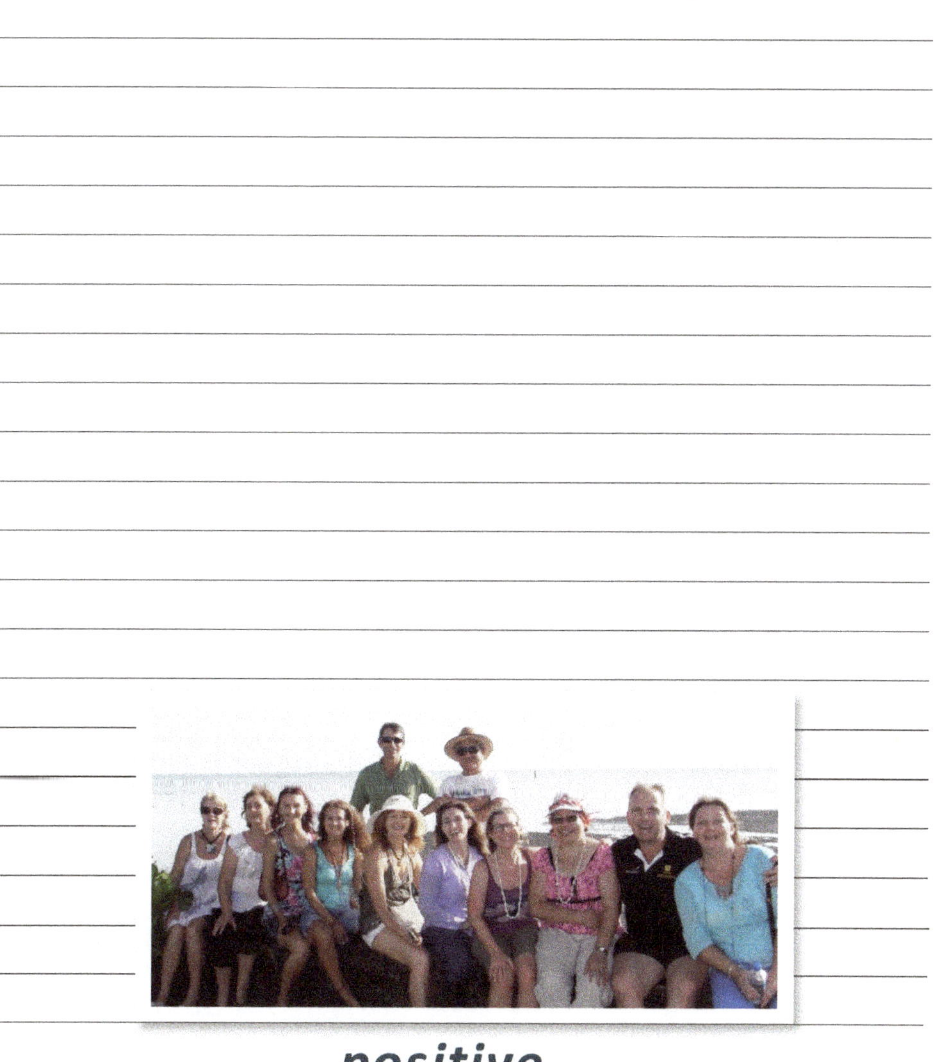

positive
AFFIRMATION

Love is all we are

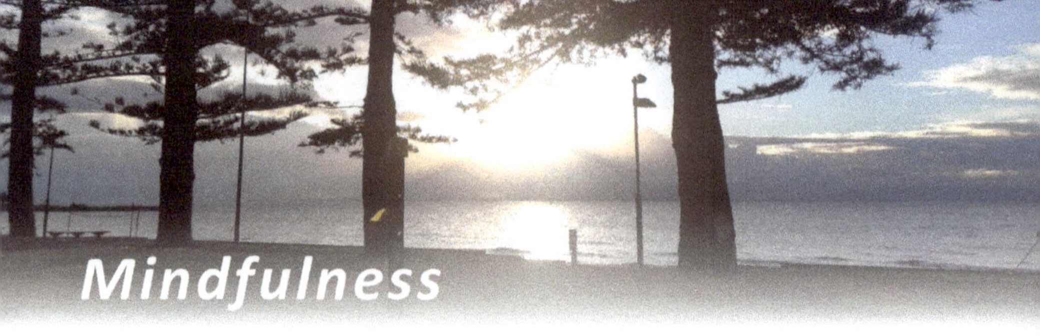

Mindfulness

Mindfulness is keeping your attention on the present moment

Whenever your thoughts take you to an anxious or negative place, take a deep breath and pay attention to the present moment. Become aware of what you see, hear, smell and taste; this will reduce worry and raise peace. Stay focused on something positive until the negative shifts. This will give you the space to see things in a more positive light.

Task: Every hour, take one minute to take deep breaths and focus on something around you that can be uplifting or positive.
You will be amazed at how much better the world looks.

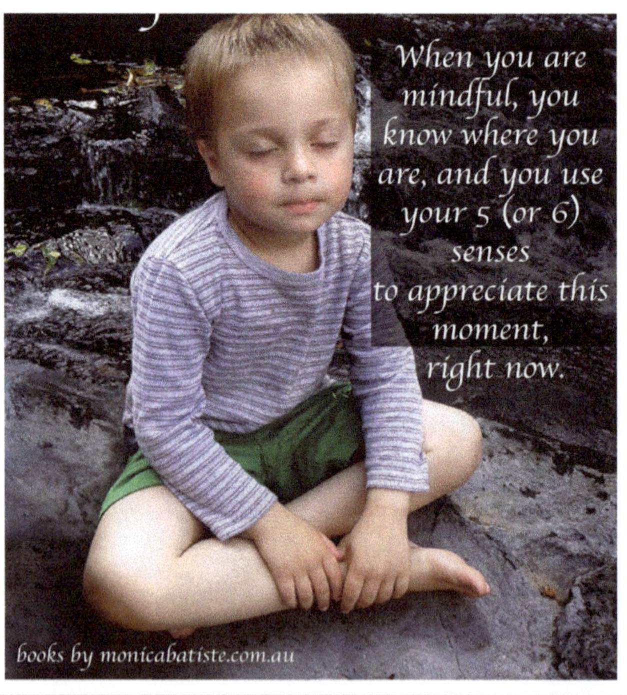

Happiness

Happiness isn't about being joyful every minute; it's about knowing you have the power to move life in the direction of your choice.

Being happy isn't about having lots of things. Although things give us pleasure, real happiness is a daily practise of being present, experiencing the moment, accepting things are as they are, being grateful for what you have, being grateful for what is to come, and focusing on the best in every situation.

Appreciation is the highest vibration. You can appreciate your family, yourself, your lifestyle and what is around you.

Allow yourself to be empowered by taking steps to make healthy choices with your self, your family, your work, your relationships, and everything in between.

When you are in alignment, you create intentions for what you want. Intend to create a life for yourself that serves you, serves the world and brings about the peace and harmony we all deserve.

Grow on a daily basis. Love yourself and others.
Trust yourself. Live with intuition.

Feel gratitude for every breath, every person, every thing, every creature and every smile that comes into your pathway.

Begin a gratitude diary. Every day write down ten things you are grateful for. This will increase your positive attitude and help open your heart to the good in life.

**When you are mindful,
you naturally release
stress and increase peace.**

CAMEL POSE

Camel pose opens the heart, flexes the spine and expands the rib cage (allowing you to take deeper breaths)

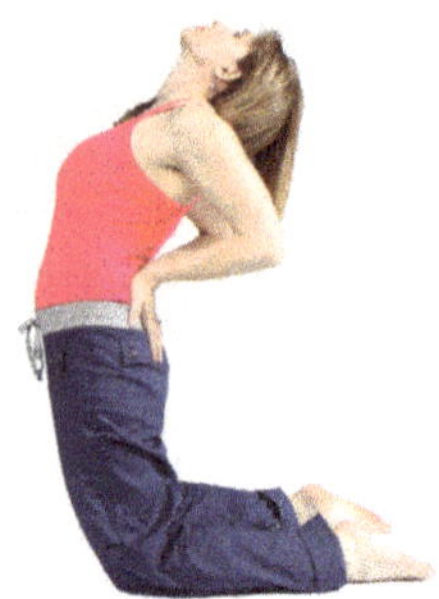

Option 1: Kneel on the floor with your knees hip width apart and thighs perpendicular to the floor. Rotate thighs inward slightly and firm but don't harden buttocks. Imagine that you're drawing your sitting bones up, into your torso. Press shins and feet firmly into floor. Rest hands on the back of your pelvis, fingers pointing down. Use your hands to spread the pelvis and lengthen it down through your tailbone. Lean back, squeeze shoulder blades together and lift heart to the sky.

Stay here for several breaths, relaxing heart and lifting torso. If there is pain in the neck, straighten head rather than leaning back.

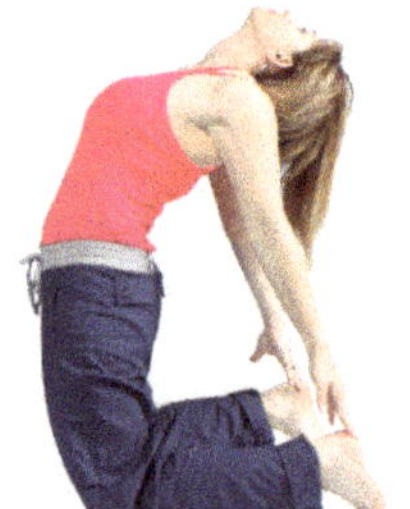

Option 2: Lift feet onto toes and reach either one hand to foot and hold for several breaths changing arms or rest fingertips onto heels and hold for several breaths.

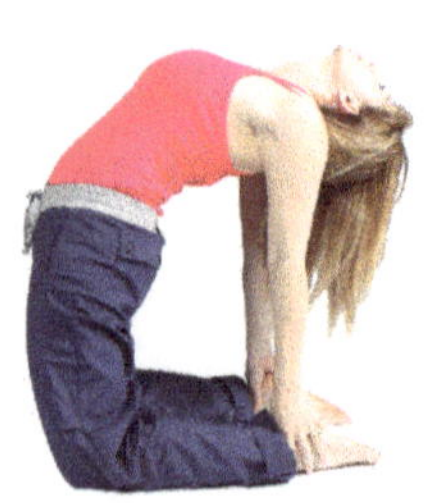

Option 3: Flatten feet to floor and ease into *Camel* by lifting hips, arching back, opening heart, squeezing shoulder blades together. Stay for several breaths. When coming out of *Camel* pose, lift head first, bring hands to lower back (as in *Soft Camel)* and move into *Child's pose,* followed by *Rabbit's pose* to allow spine to stretch, recover and relax.

RABBIT'S POSE

Rabbit's pose lengthens the spine and releases tension

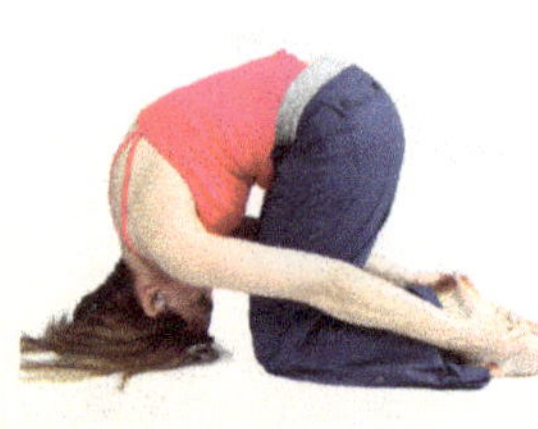

Grip heels with hands, place the crown of the head onto mat in front of knees and lift hips to sky. By lifting the hips you will feel your arms and shoulders release and the spine lengthen. Stay for several breaths and move into Child's pose to allow blood pressure to equalise before coming out.

Child's Pose

Relaxes spine and hips, helping you feel safe and happy

Keep big toes together and knees slightly apart. Bring bottom to heels and rest head on the earth. Rest arms by side, or another option of your choice.

If head is uncomfortable, rest your head on your hands. *Child's pose* is a relaxing and recovery pose. Come to this pose to breathe and let go. Feel your body relax.

Remain here as long as you like. Breathe deeply, let shoulders melt. Breathe and relax. Let go of tension.

Send yourself love messages,

you are already perfect, beautiful and lovable.

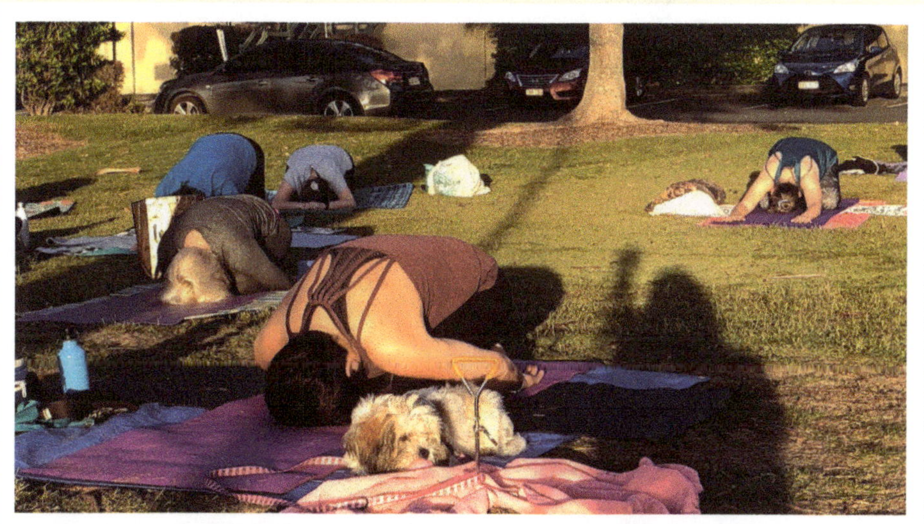

❀ ❀ ❀

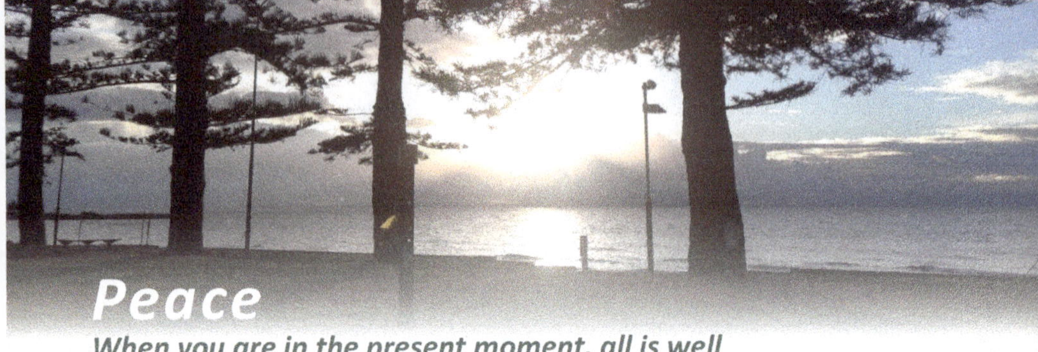

Peace

When you are in the present moment, all is well

Yoga encourages you to let go of expectations, blame, shame and comparisons. You are encouraged to love, honour and accept yourself, just as you are, right now. As you learn to accept the tightness here and the holding on there, you naturally let it go. When you let it go, you relax and move forward. Yoga stretches muscles and minds. It releases long held tension in the psyche.

Going with the flow will support your breath, body, brain and circumstances.

Breathe. Let go. You've got this. You can do this. You're doing it now. accept. Breathe. Be mindful. Be here. It is okay. It's going to be okay.

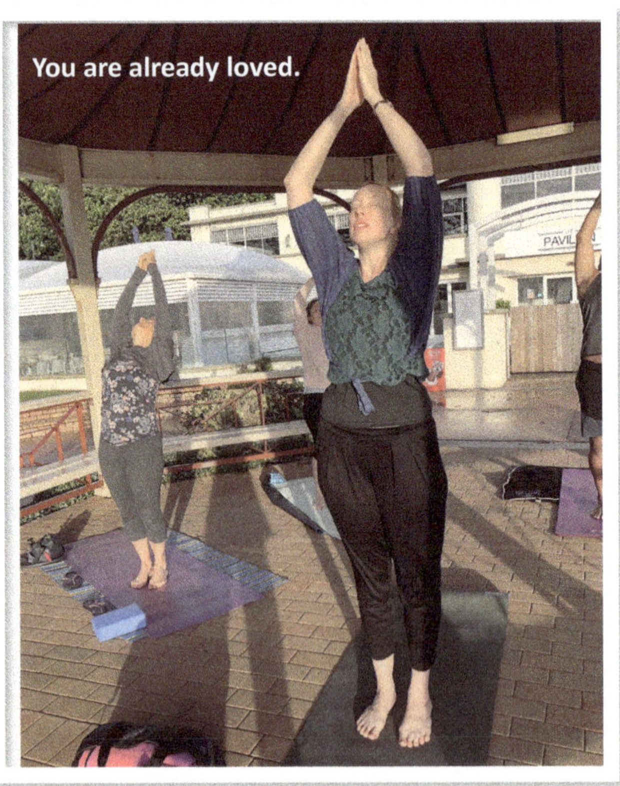

Releasing stress through yoga

Stress is a response to danger - either real or percieved

You have the power to move life in the direction of your choice.

When danger approaches, the stress response can save your life. Your heart rate will quicken, adrenaline will rise, and your muscles will pump. You will be ready to fight in one second!

Each of us learns how to respond to danger in our own way. For some, the stress response is to fight, for others it's to run away, and some people freeze, please or faint.

This is your survival strategy when facing danger, but what if there is no danger, you just 'think' there is, or your responding to a triggered danger response.

In the stress response, you will respond the same as when facing real danger - but there will be no release. You aren't going to fight your boss, run away from a client, or stop and hide, even if you want to.

When we feel stress without release, we develop coping strategies. Eventually this stress can damage your body, and erode your joy for life.

Recognising and releasing the stress response

When you notice your breath is shorter and your heart rate higher, your stress response is being triggered. You may notice your sense of awareness changes too, you might have a heightened sense of what is happening around you if you switch on fight or flight, but if you switch on freeze – you may feel a dulling of your senses.

As soon as you notice the stress response, focus on deep breaths. Lower your diaphragm to give more room to your breath. Deep breaths are a signal to your body that you are safe. Breathe deeply no matter what is going on around you. Relax your tummy and hips. Let go through the hip flexors. Continue to breathe and become present by connecting to the earth, noticing the sky (even if it's in your imagination) and visualising something peaceful. Clients won't notice. The traffic won't change. Your partner will keep talking, but you will be clearer. For a simple guide to breathing; breathe in for six seconds, and breathe out for six seconds. Soon you will shift, and the world will become clearer.

Yoga switches on peace with deep breathing, mindfulness and meditation. As you learn to let go inside yoga, you learn to let go in life.

You are worthy and deserving of a happy life

forgiveness

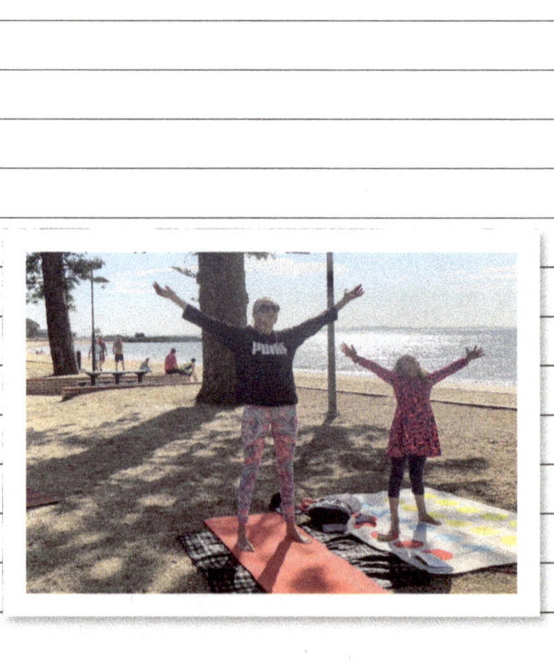

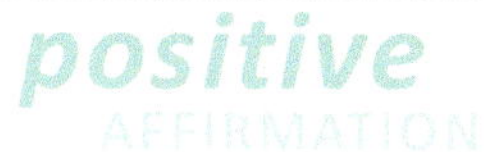

I am already lovable, just as I am

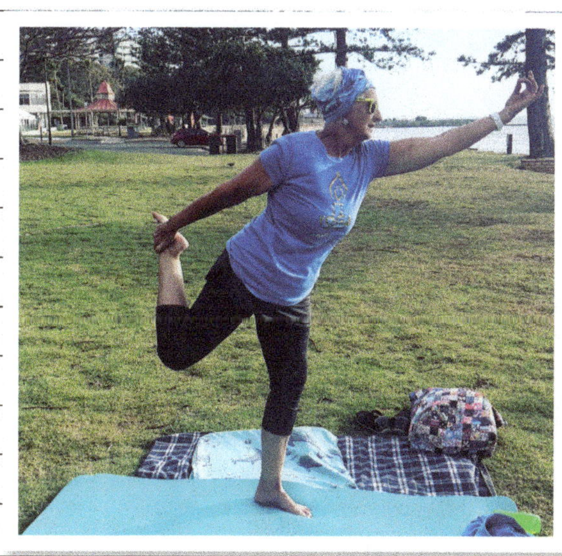

positive
AFFIRMATION

I let go of negative patterns and embrace the positive

self-love

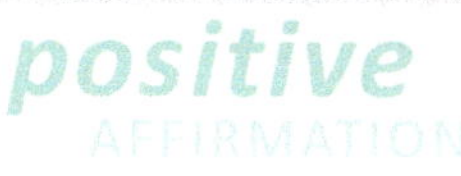

positive
AFFIRMATION

I am playful

acceptance

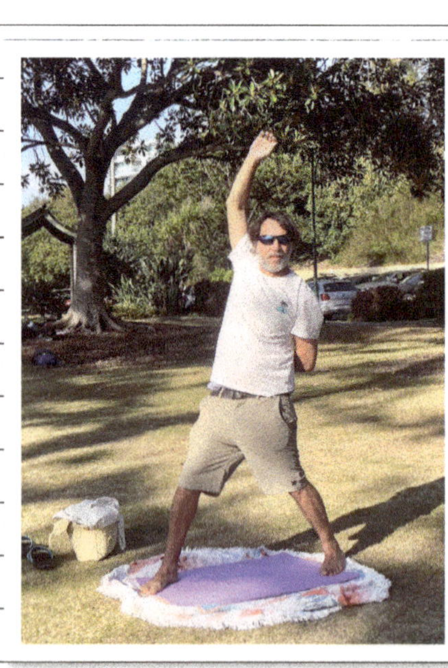

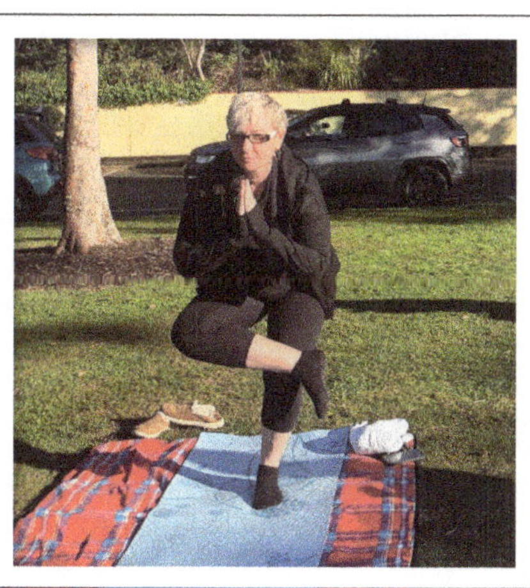

Emotional intelligence Self-Esteem

Yoga helps you grow emotional intelligence and intuition, because yoga teaches you about yourself.

Yoga is an extension of life's moments. During yoga all virtues can be acknowledged, for each posture expresses a virtue, and virtues grow emotional intelligence.

We have a natural ability to love and accept ourselves; all we need to do is allow ourselves to grow what is already there.

If you can acknowledge and be gentle with yourself, you will find yourself growing happier and more resilient each day.

Parents teach emotional intelligence through role modelling, and positive reinforcement. Positive reinforcement is naming the virtue your child is demonstrating. Every time you name the virtue, the virtue within that child grows.

For example, when you see your child being peaceful, your first reaction might be to have a break. But if you can first say to your child, 'I see your peacefulness right now,' you have taught him/her that what they are doing in that moment is called peacefulness. Acknowledge peace again and again... and soon your child develops the recognition of what peace looks like, how to get there, and that they can be peaceful.

The next time you need to call your child to peace, they are right there. Because they know it, they've heard you acknowledge it, and they know what it means.

Acknowledging your own virtues is tricky at first, especially if you're used to criticism. Begin with journaling and writing about your day. Look through your notes and find your virtues. 'I see my kindness here, and my strength there. I was generous here, and forgiving there.'. You already exhibit hundreds of virtues a day, and from this moment on, commit to finding your self-esteem and growing into the person you were born to be.

Acknowledgment starts right here, wherever you are, and when you acknowledge virtues during everyday life, you see the transformation of yours and your child's self-esteem. When your child makes the connection that they can self regulate their own emotions, they will thrive.

As adults and children grow self-esteem, they will take charge of how they feel, even when they are faced with tough situations. Resilience grows from self-esteem, and it is important because the higher the resilience, the easier it is to recover from setbacks.

For instance, if someone is faced with defeat, fails an exam, is rejected from their dream job or partner, the first response is going to be disappointment, but how they respond and what they do next depends on how that person feels about themselves.

An emotionally intelligent person will acknowledge how they feel, and support themselves in a healthy way. They will understand that it hurts, know it will eventually pass, not blame themselves, and as the hurt subsides, they will resume actions to achieve their goals. They will still believe in themselves.

The low self-esteem person feels defeated. They might see this as one more piece of evidence that they are a failure, that they cannot achieve, that this is probably their fault. They are likely to feel powerless and helpless, and use negative words to describe their situation. Without emotional intelligence they cannot successfully move through pain or overcome difficulty.

Without resilience, some people will turn to sulking, anger or depression. They might change the way they deal with life permanently in order to resist the chances of being rejected in the future.

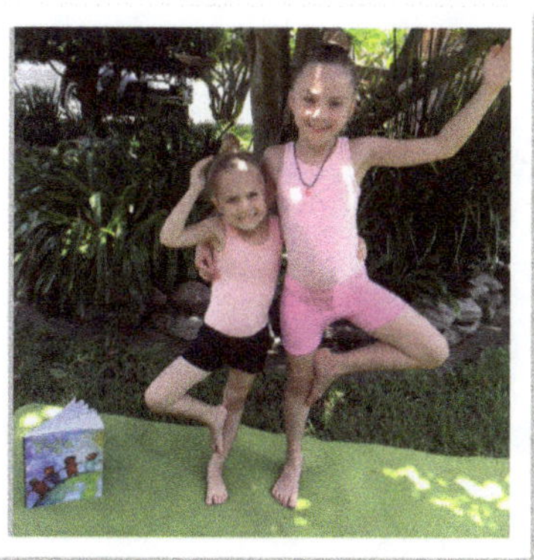

An emotionally intelligent person will acknowledge how they feel, and support themselves in a healthy way.

Low self-esteem can be the trigger for mental health and substance abuse.

Your mental health is the most important aspect of role modelling for yourself and your family. If you are looking after you, your child will copy that. If you are loving you, they will love themselves. If you are demonstrating kindness and caring towards yourself, then so will your child.
It's all about you. Love, honour and accept yourself right now, and move forward with gentleness and kindness.

Acknowledge your own successes and achievements, no matter how small, and then you will automatically do this with your child, and he or she will automatically do it for themselves and others.

Every day in every way, life is getting better and better and better.

Growing Self-Esteem
I see you

*Naming the virtues you see in yourself and your children
is the building blocks of self-esteem.*

Yoga is the perfect platform to acknowledge character and virtues.

Acceptance
Agility
Ambition
Assertiveness
Attention
Awareness
Balance
Beauty
Benevolence
Bravery
Caring
Charity
Clarity
Cleanliness
Commitment
Compassion
Communication
Confidence
Concentration
Considerate
Consistent
Co-operation
Courage
Courtesy

Creativity
Curiosity
Dependability
Detachment
Determination
Dedication
Decisiveness
Desire

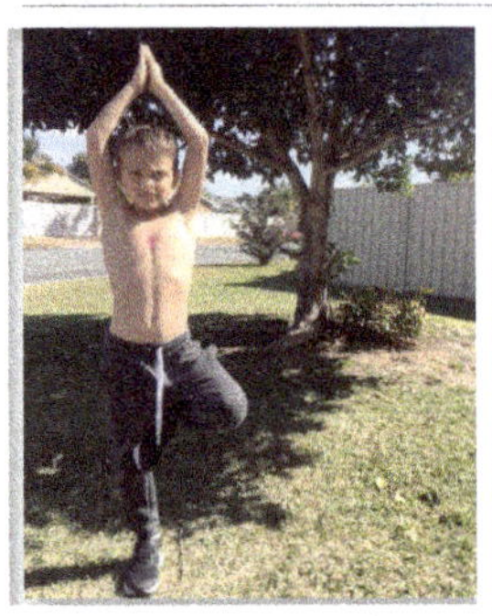

Discernment
Discretion
Discipline
Divergent-thinking
Empathy
Energy
Enthusiasm
Ethics

Eloquence
Excellence
Expand comfort-zone
Exponential
Faith
Flexibility
Focus
Forgiveness
Friendliness
Friendship
Fun
Generosity
Gentleness
Grace
Gratitude
Grounded
Happiness
Harmony
Health
Heroic
Helpfulness
Honesty
Honour
Hope

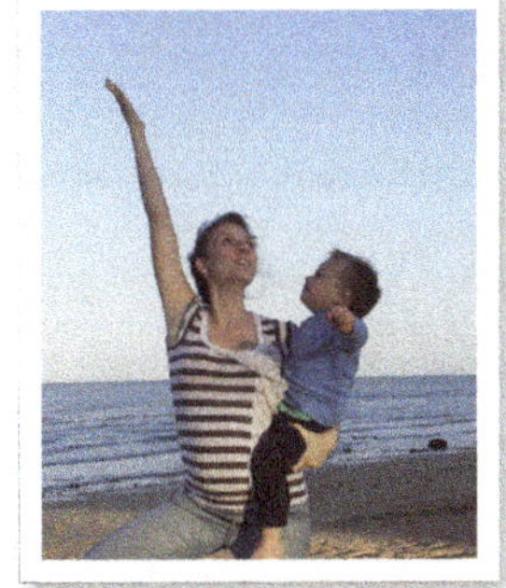

Humility

Humour

Imagination

Integrity

Initiative

Idealism

Innocence

Intuition

Joyful

Justice

Jovial

Kindness

Leadership

Letting-go

Logical

Love

Loyalty

Manners

Meditation

Mindfulness

Mercy

Moderation

Modesty

Motivation

Negotiation

Open-Heart

Optimism

Orderliness

Patience

Peacefulness

Perseverance

Playful

Positive

Purposefulness

Reliability

Reparation

Resilience

Respect

Responsibility

Reverence

Self-Awareness

Self-Belief

Self-Care

Self-Confidence

Self-Discipline

Self-Esteem

Self-Love

Self-Reliance

Self-Respect

Self-Regulation

Service

Social-Skills

Spiritual

Steadfastness

Strength

Sincerity

Tact

Tenderness

Thankfulness

Tolerance

Trust

Truthfulness

Unity

Understanding

Values

Visionary

Wholistic

Wisdom

Wonder

Zealous

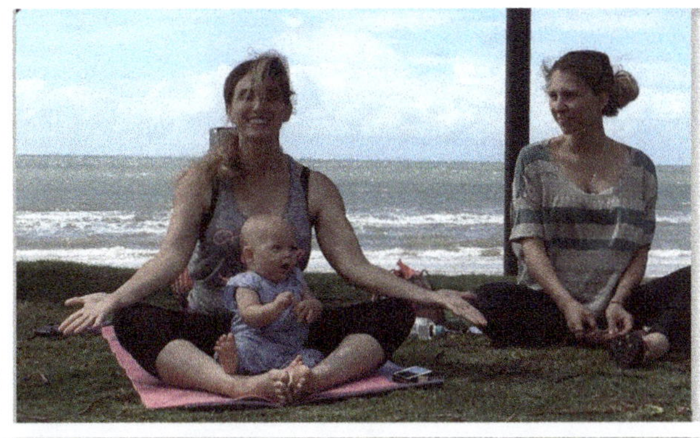

self-acceptance

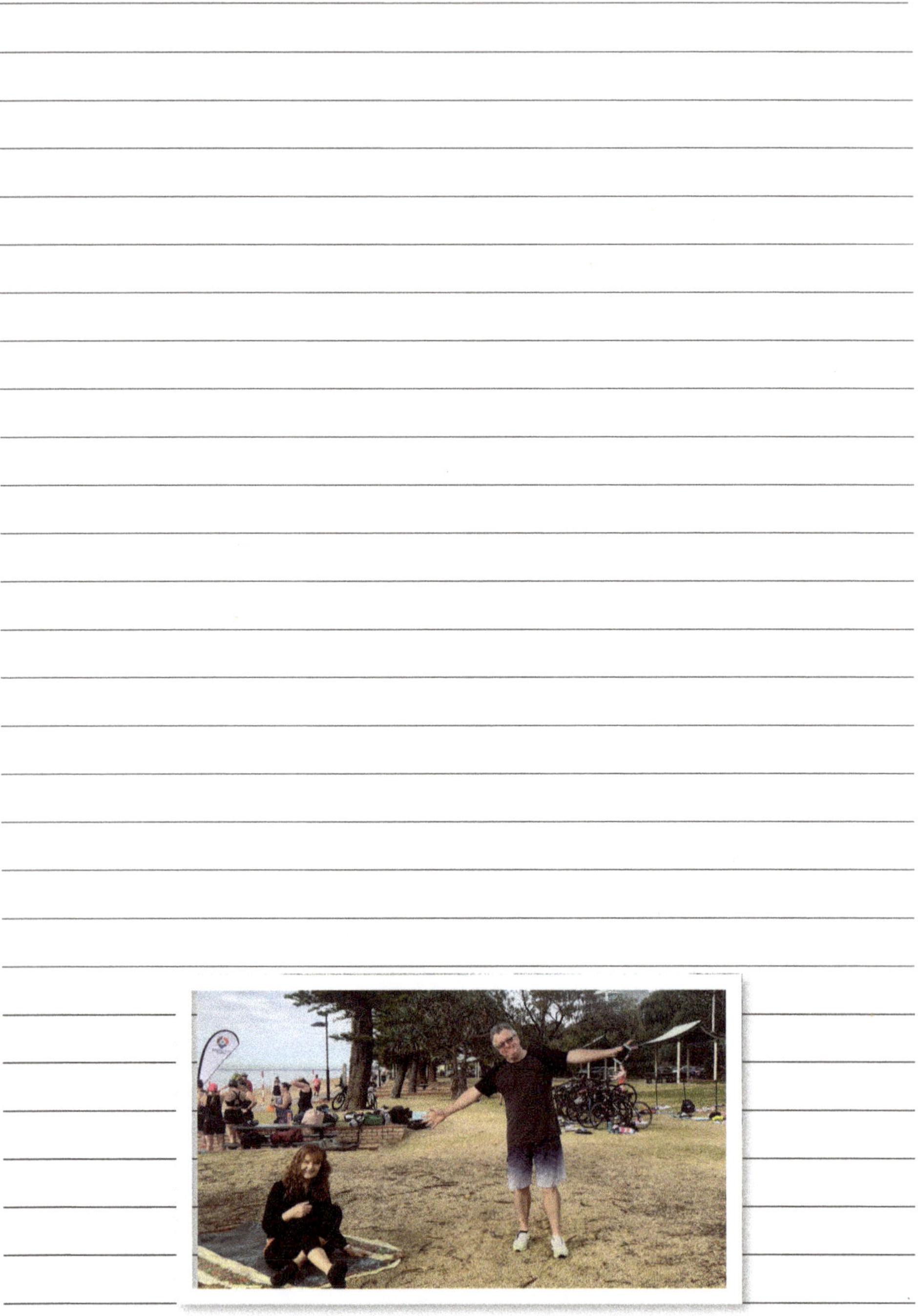

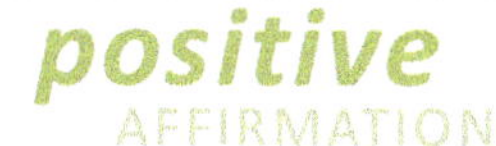

positive
AFFIRMATION

I am already perfect, just as i am

beauty

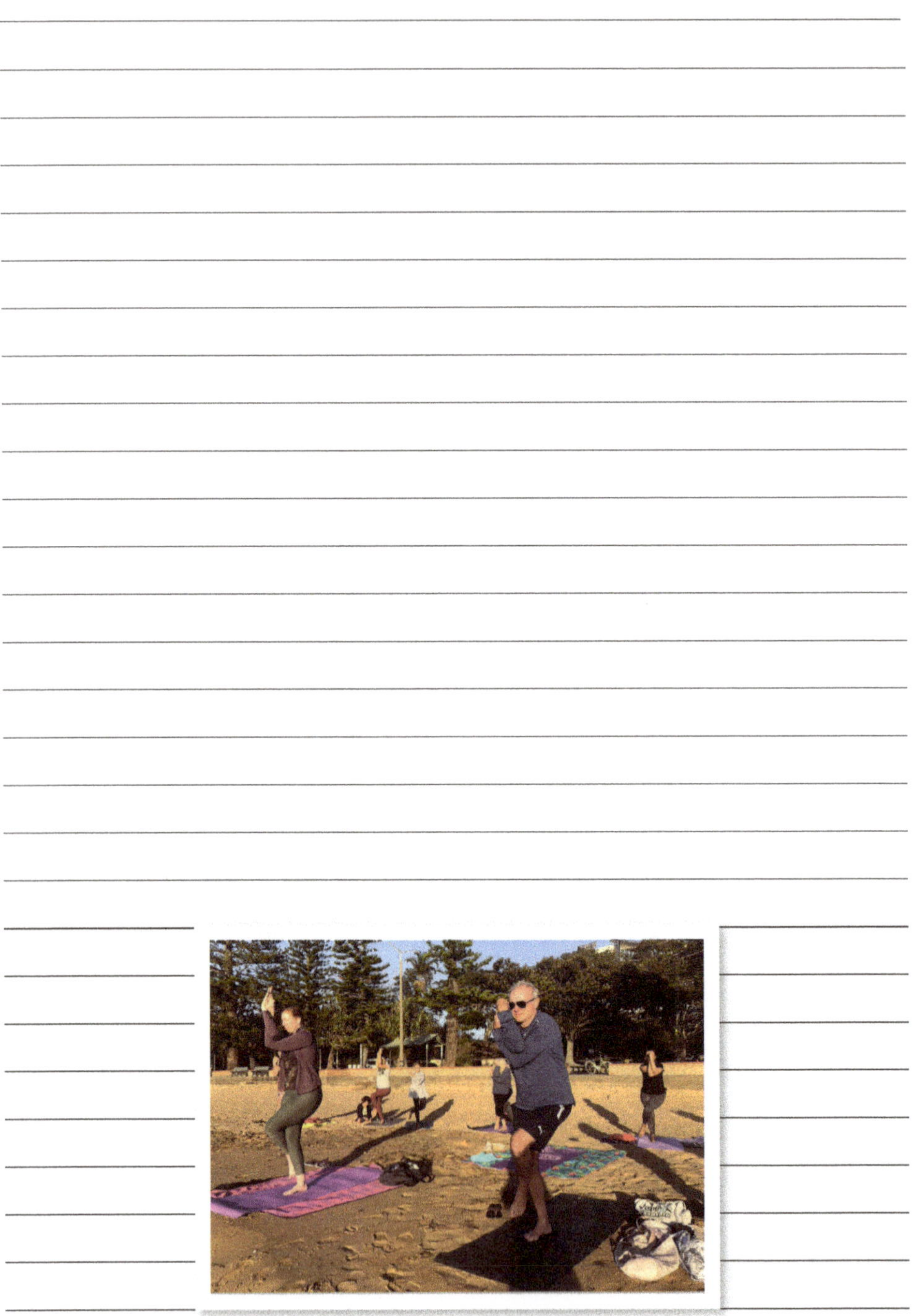

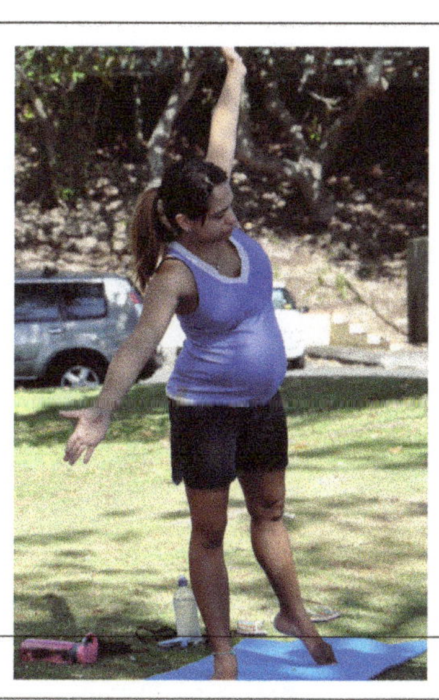

positive

AFFIRMATION

I am strong and beautiful

perserverance

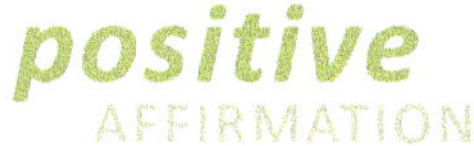

positive
AFFIRMATION

I trust myself

intuition

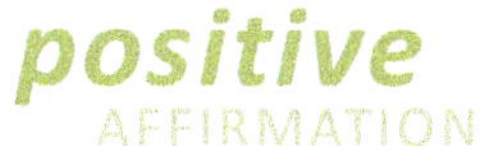

I am assertive confident and I believe in me

Self-esteem for all ages

Reinforcement of virtues in character

Support your child's character by naming virtues.
Some examples

'I see your flexibility and focus.'

That must have taken some determination.'

'I see your joy.'

'Thank you for your kindness'

'I noticed your strength'
'That took courage.'

Support your child's character by guiding their virtues

'It's going to take commitment for you to achieve that.'

You can do this.
You are already doing this.
Well done.

'I trust you.'

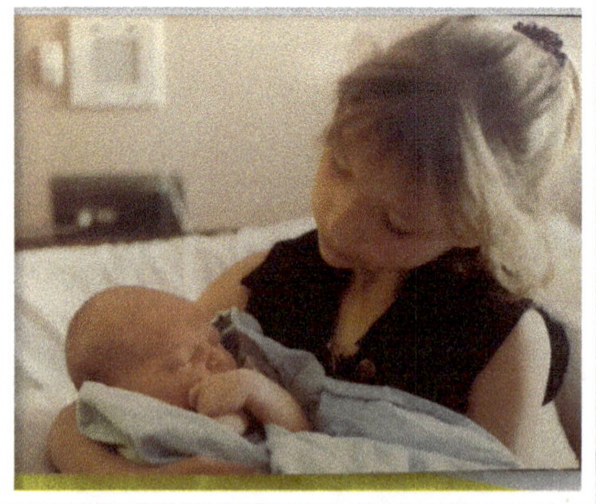

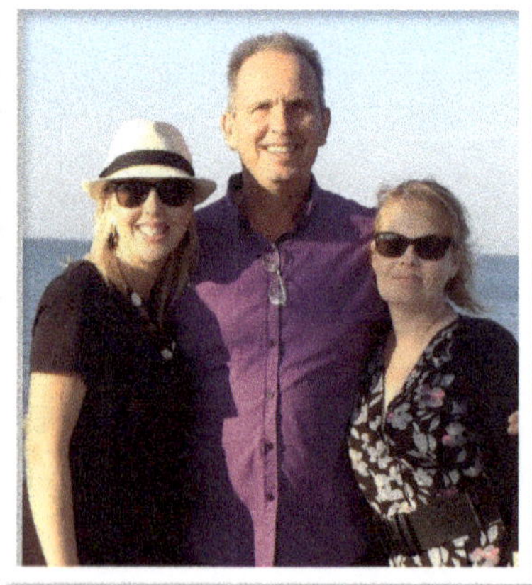

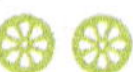

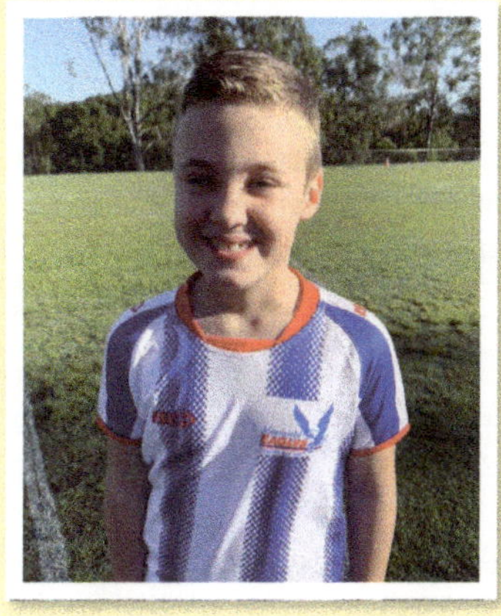

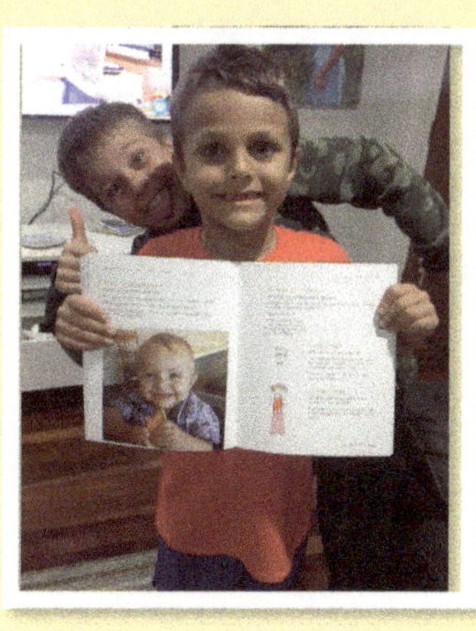

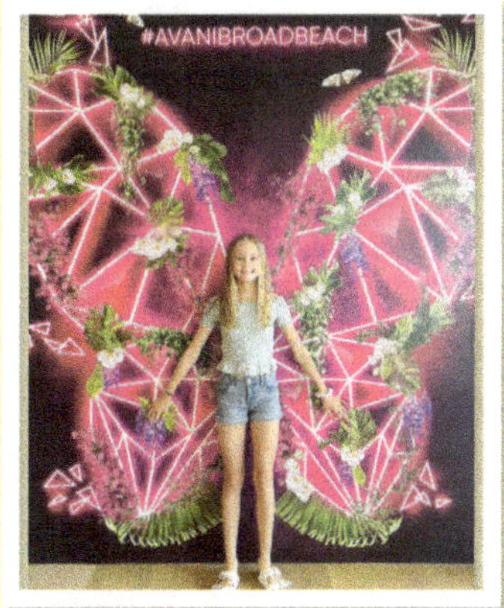

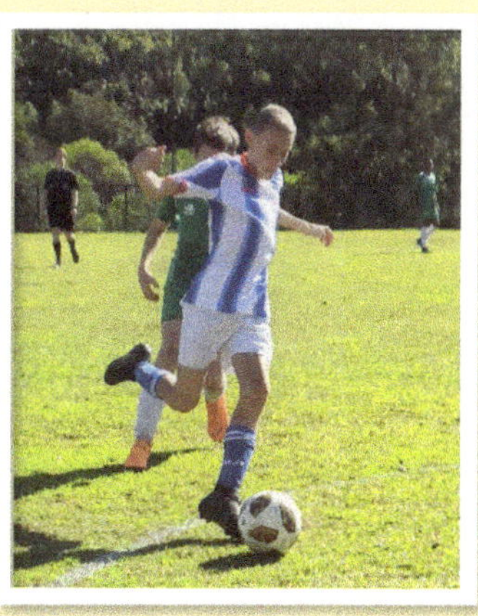

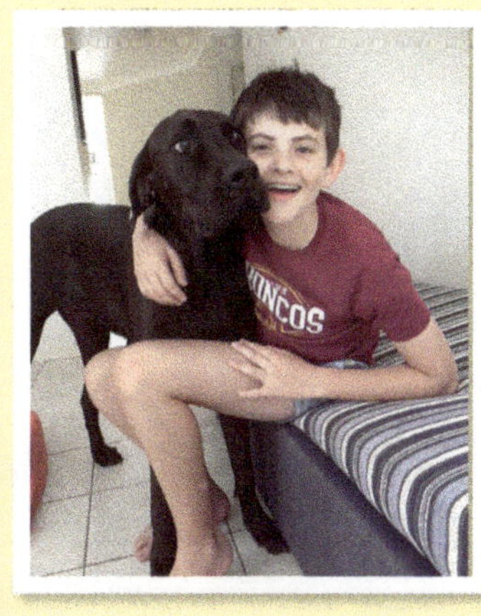

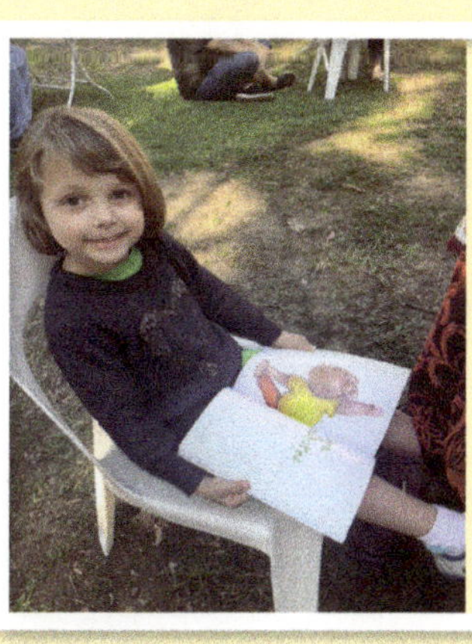

F
A
M
I
L
Y

WARRIOR POSES

Warrior poses help to grow strength, courage, flexibility and balance

Warrior Poses are for confidence, grounding and courage.
With your heart open and your arms ready for action, Warrior poses help you reach your goals with enthusiasm and self-belief.

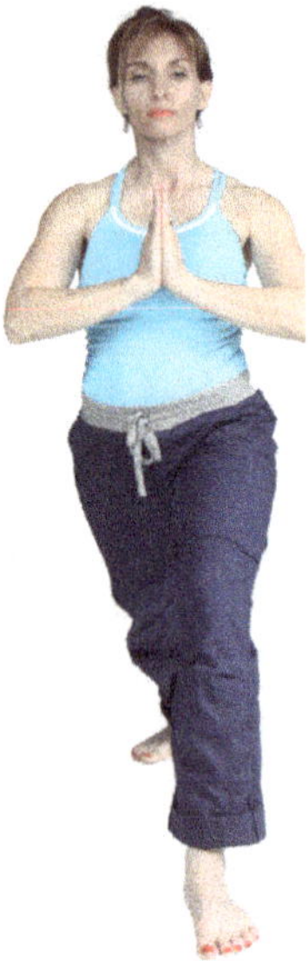

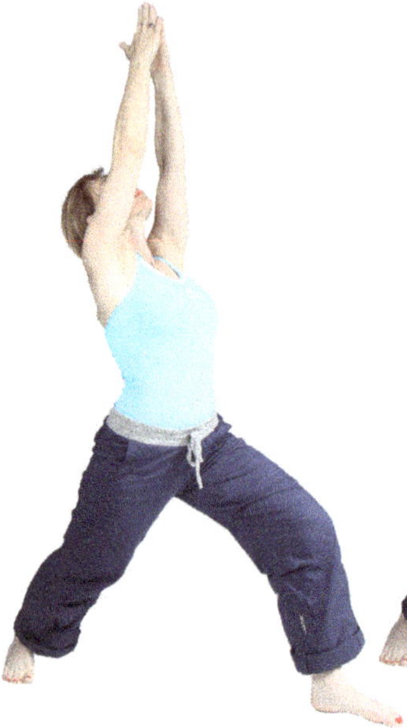

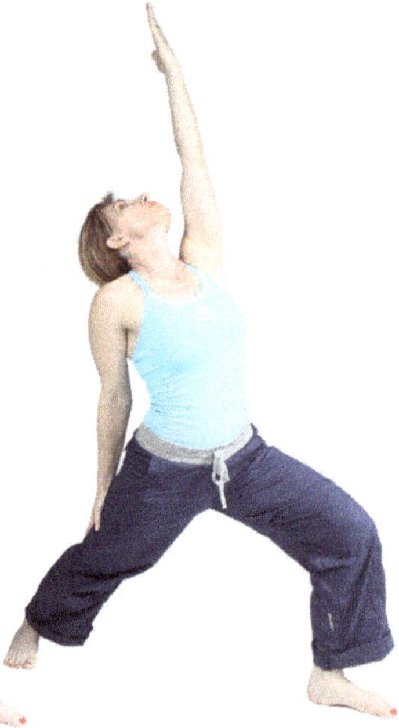

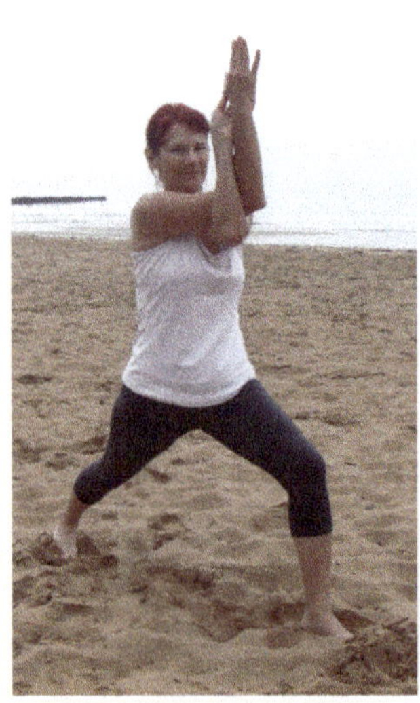

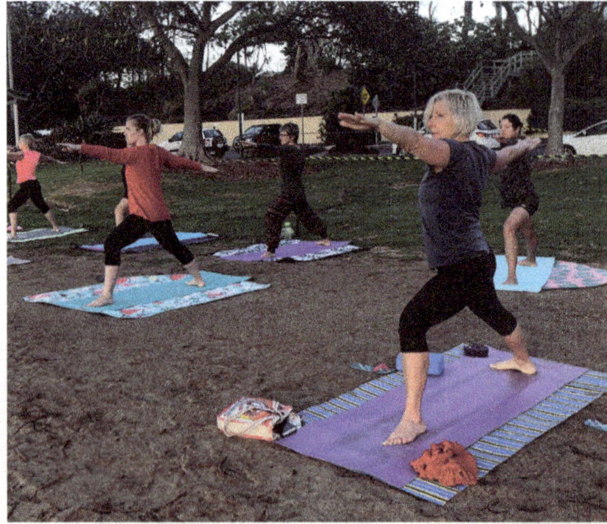

WARRIOR POSES
variations and adaptations

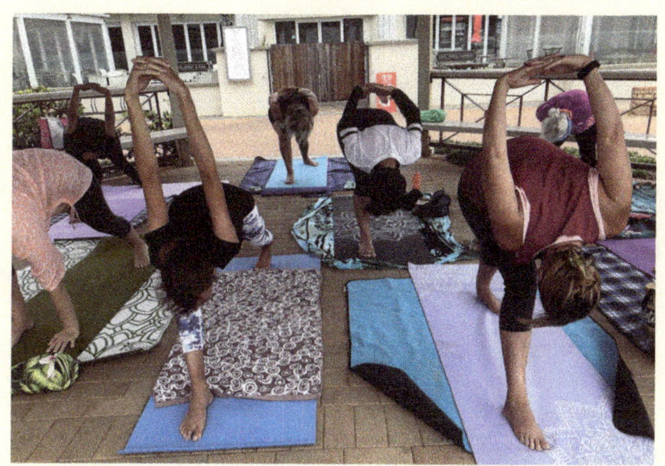

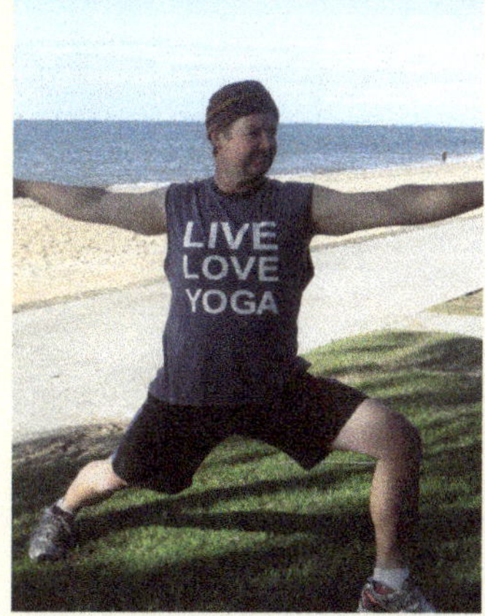

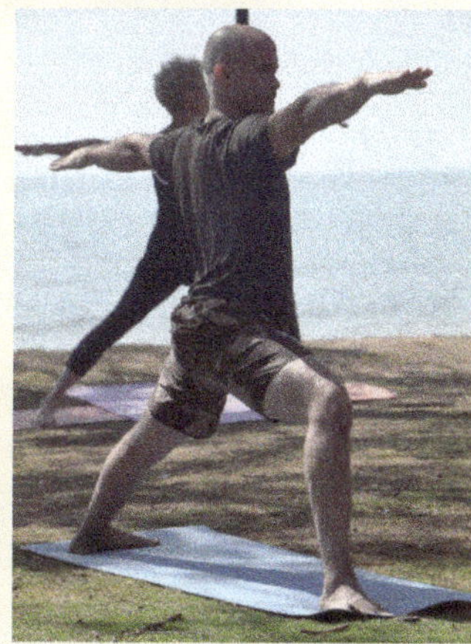

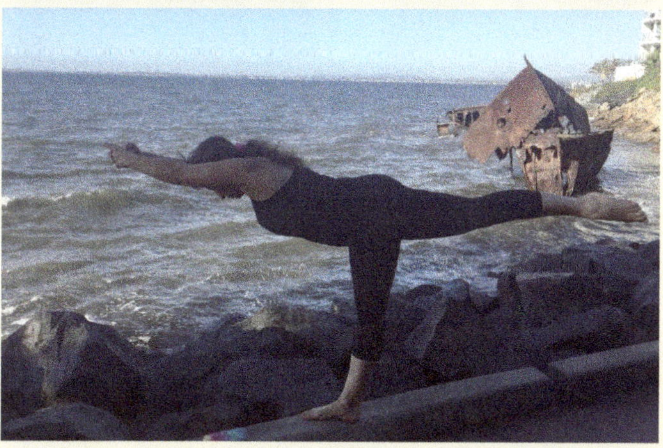

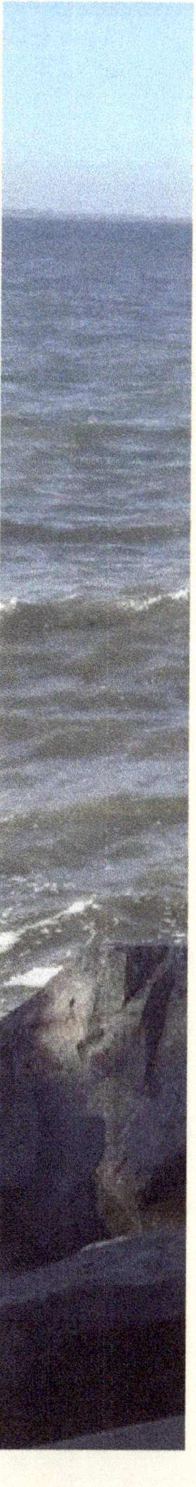

Learn and Grow

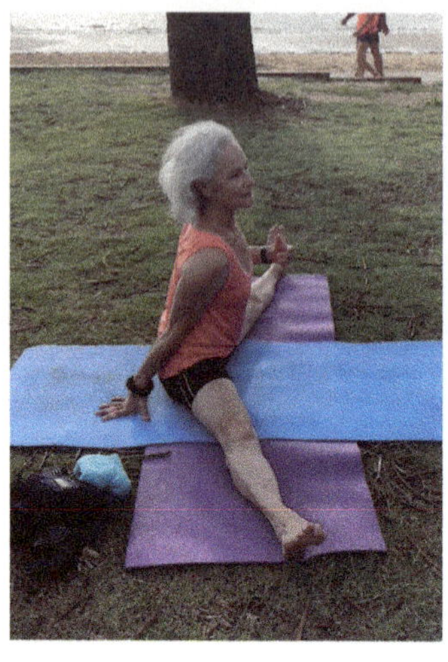 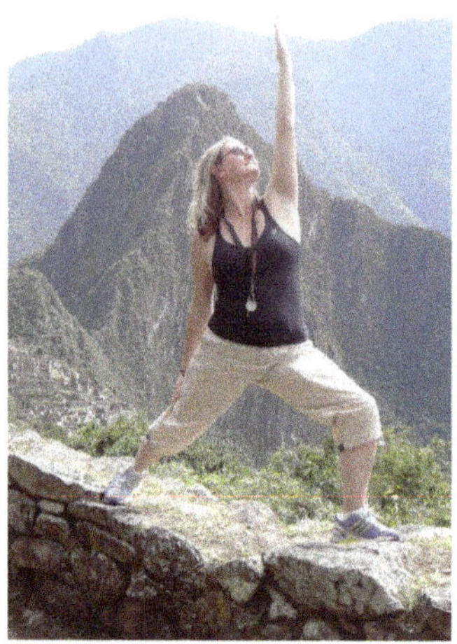

Every day in every way, better and better and better

Expand yourself by trying all the different kinds of yoga classes and teachers. Seek new experiences and learn as much as you can. By doing this, you will grow, expand and thrive.

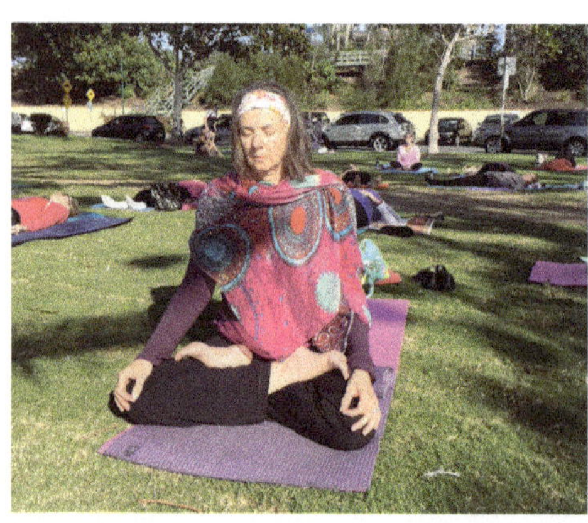 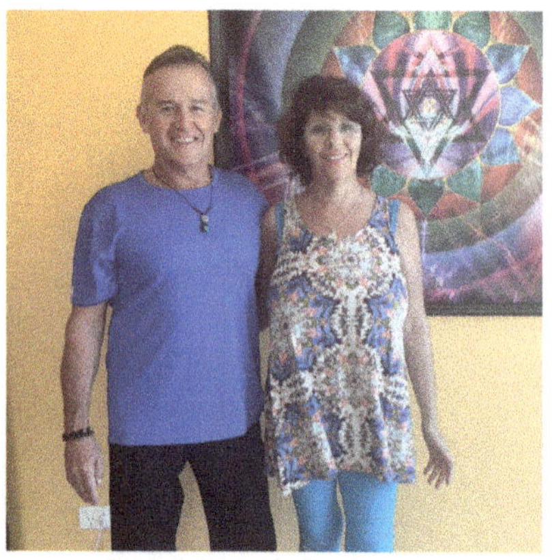

Yoga is for every-one and every-body

Breathe   Balance   Focus   Believe

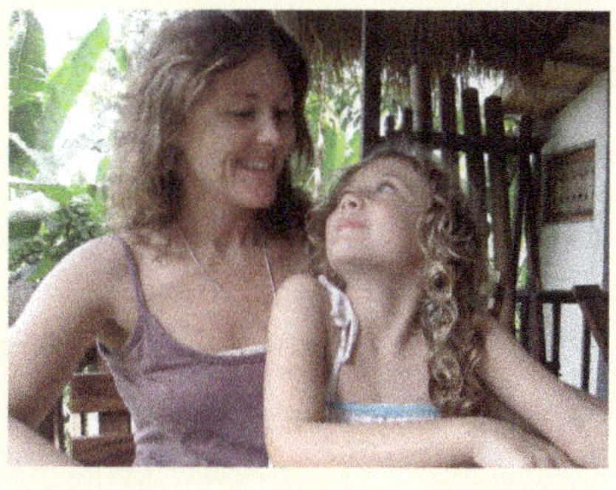

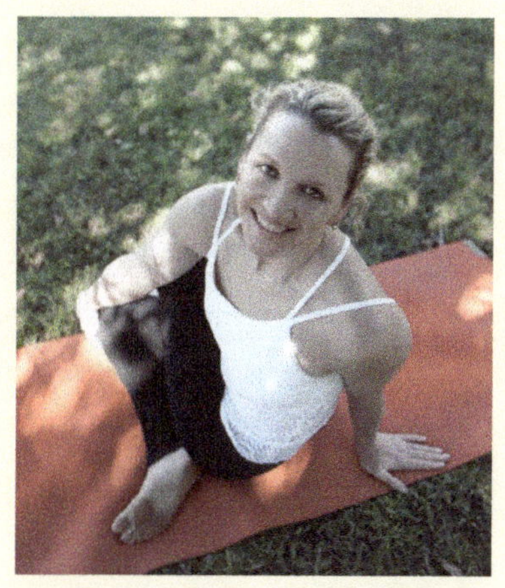

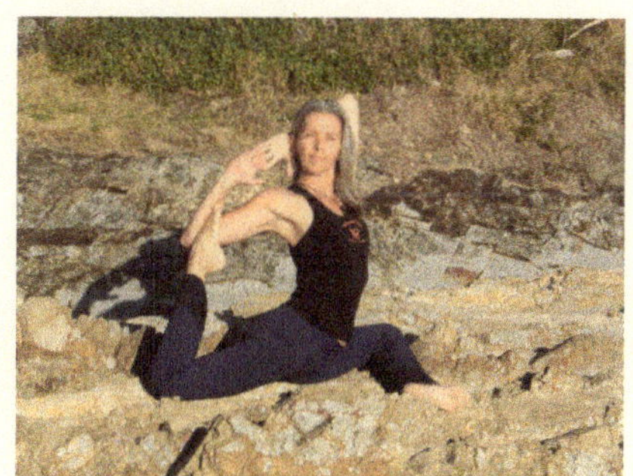

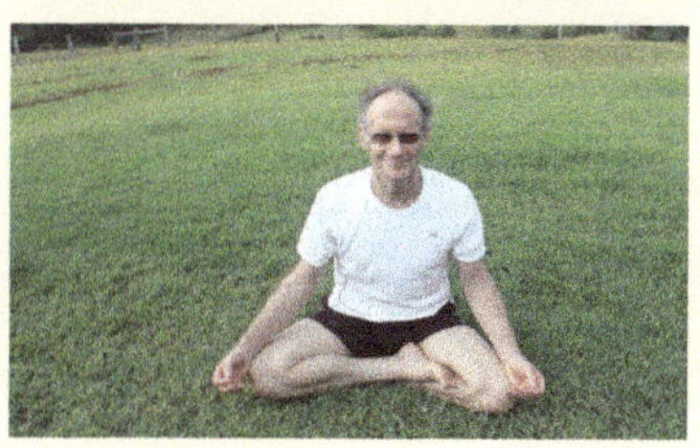

Love

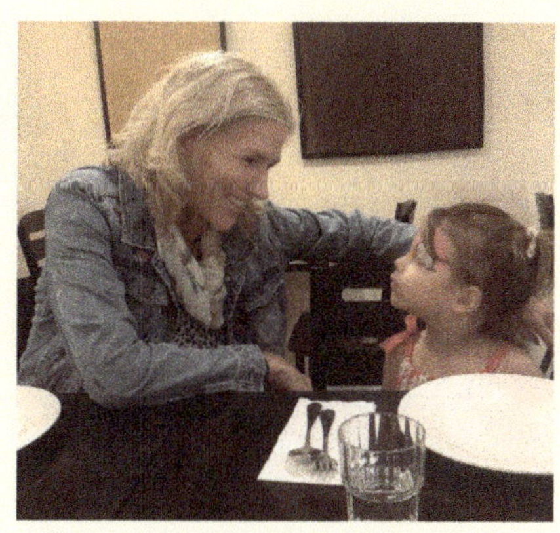

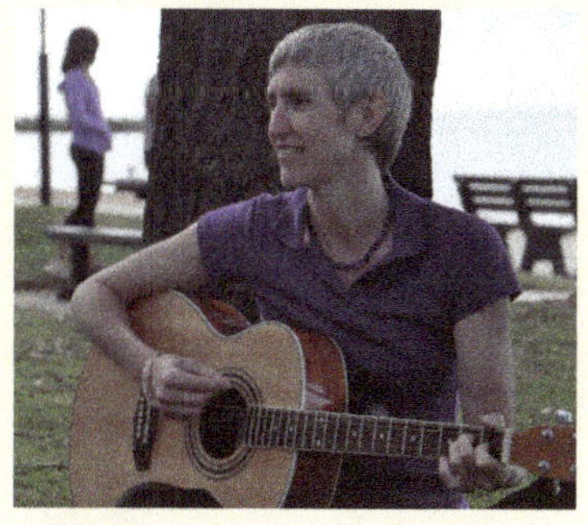

Love honour and accept yourself, just as you are

commitment

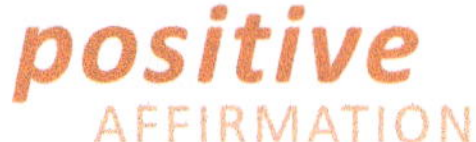

positive
AFFIRMATION

I am empowered, and I create my wonderful life

compassion

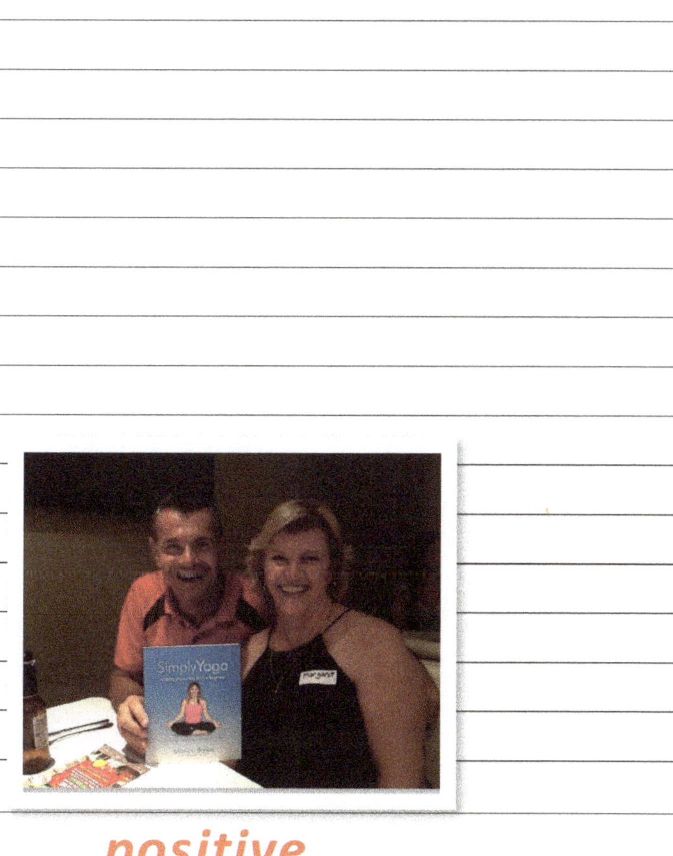

positive
AFFIRMATION

I send love ahead to where ever I go

flexible

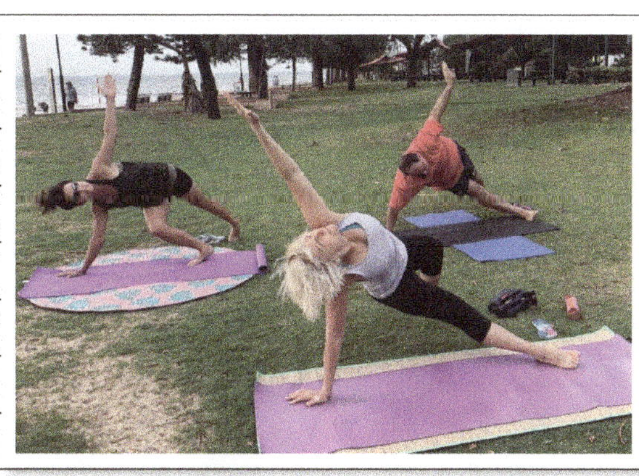

positive
AFFIRMATION

I take loving care of myself

hope

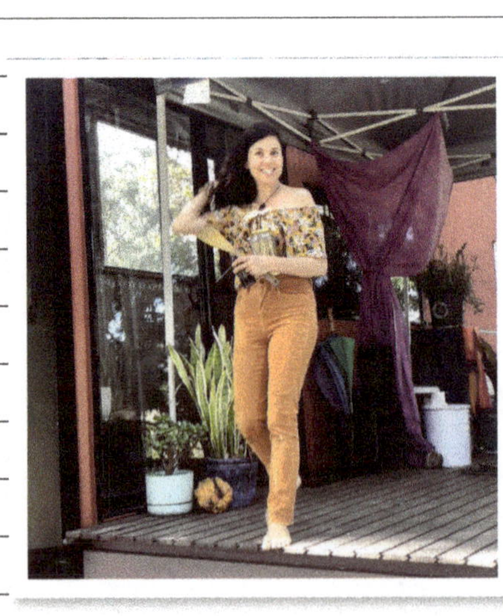

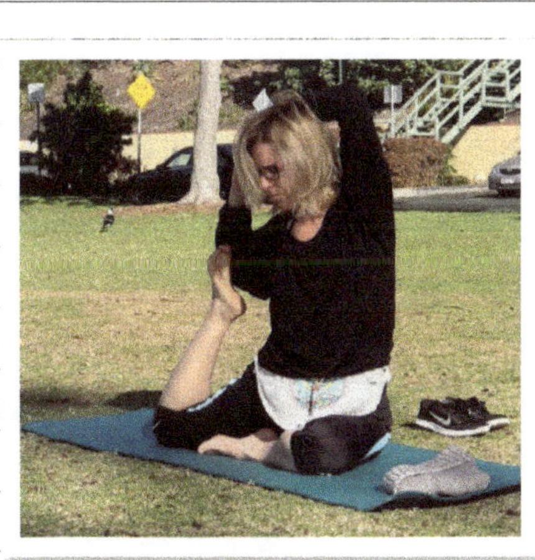

positive
AFFIRMATION

I embrace life

PIGEON POSE

Pigeon pose is an excellent pose to help prevent or relieve sciatica
Pigeon pose releases the piriformis in the gluteus, which is the muscle that tightens around the sciatic nerve. *Pigeon pose* opens the hips, lenthens the ITB band, and lengthens the hip flexor on the lower leg.

From *Downward Dog*, lift one leg and rotate the hip up toward the sky. for *Three Legged Dog.*

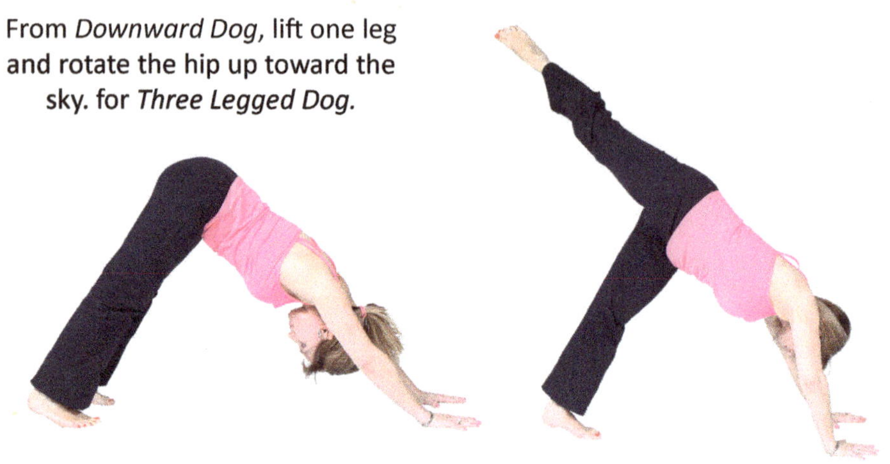

From *Three Legged Dog*, scoop top leg through and rest it across the mat.
Rotate hips to bring them parallel to the mat.
Pigeon pose Option one, stay on hands, option two, fold onto arms and option three, lay on the mat with outstretched arms. Press heart onto mat to open groin. Relax and breathe into tight muscles. Let go of pain.
Breathe into the peace of *Pigeon pose* for up to one minute. Lengthen through the body with extended arms for a stronger option. If there is any pain in your knee, roll over towards your hip to take off pressure, or onto your back for *Hip Opener.*

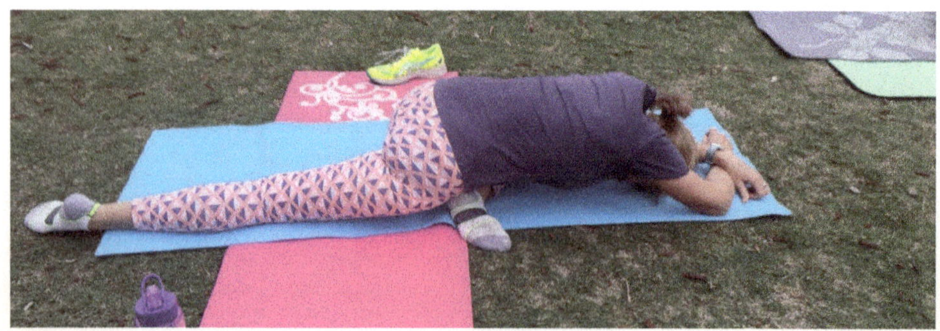

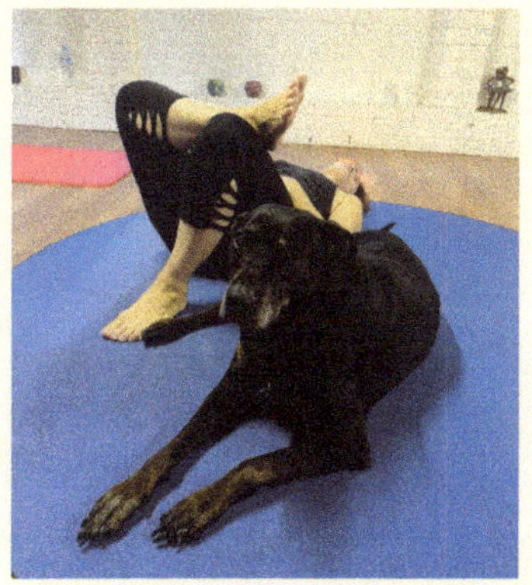

HIP OPENER

If *Pigeon pose* is too strong, roll onto your back and do a *Hip-Opener* instead. Cross right foot over left knee, place right hand onto right inner thigh and press until you feel the stretch through the hip. Hold for 1 - 2 minutes. Change sides.

TWISTED PIGEON

A fun twist from *Pigeon pose* is *Twisted Pigeon*. It's like *Thread the Needle* meets *Pigeon*. Twist away from the open hip to extend the opening. From *Pigeon pose*, rise to your hands, lift the opposite hand to foot and slip through to *Thread the Needle*. Lengthen the arm away and readjust shoulders. The other arm can stay pressed for option one, lift towards the sky for option two, or wrap around your back for option three. It's a strong posture, but feels great.

Feeling good is what it's all about, and sometimes time out is all you need to let go, and let love in.

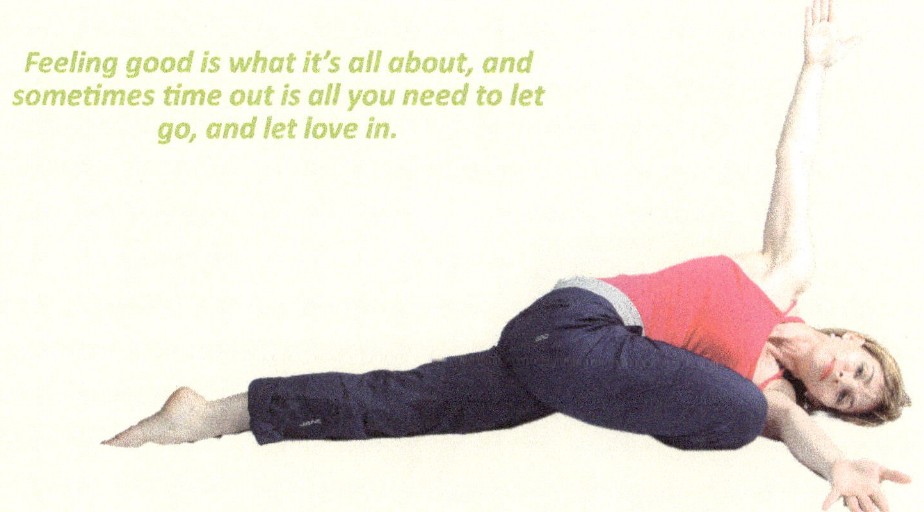

Release *Pigeon* or *Hip Opener* with a free choice. A rock through the hips, a *Downward dog, Cat-Cow,* whatever you need. It's your choice. Repeat *Pigeon* or *Hip-Opener* on other side.

PLANK POSE

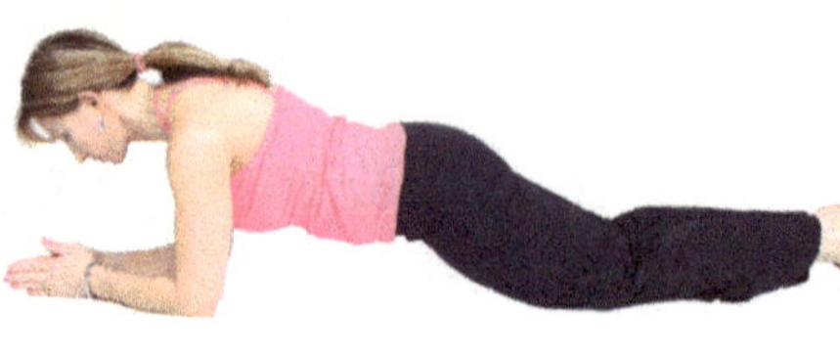

From hands and knees, choose your *Plank Pose.* For all options keep pelvic floor and belly tucked in.

Option 1: Forearms and knees, hold for up to one minute.

Option 2: Hands or forearms. Lift knees and press through the toes. 1 - 3 minutes.

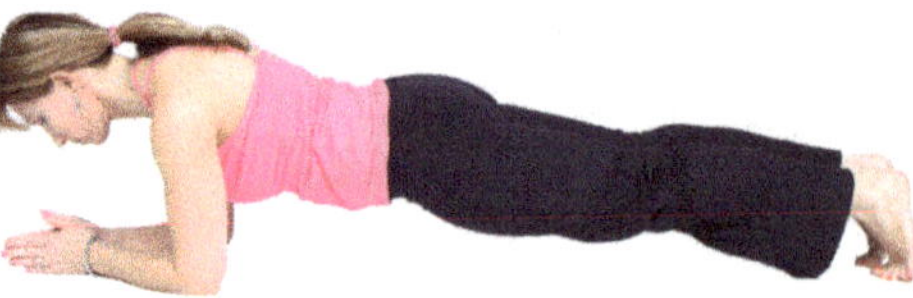

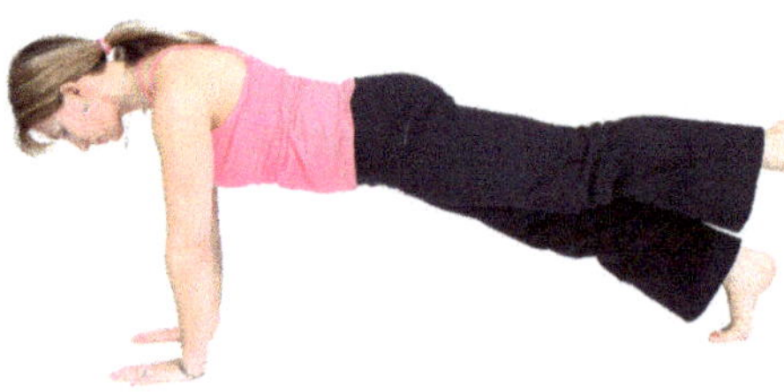

Option 3: During *Plank*, lift one leg for thirty seconds, then lift the other leg.

Option 4: Lift one leg and opposite hand for thirty seconds, change sides.

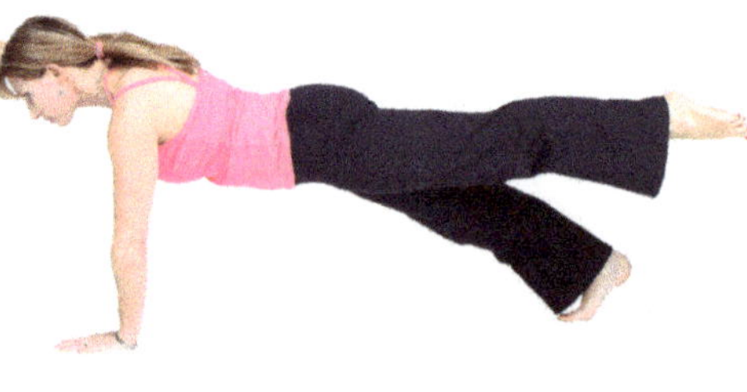

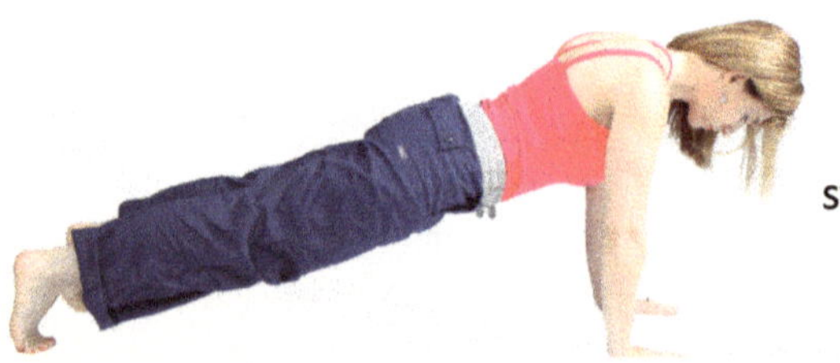

Option 5: Gradually build your strongest pose to three minutes.

Bow pose

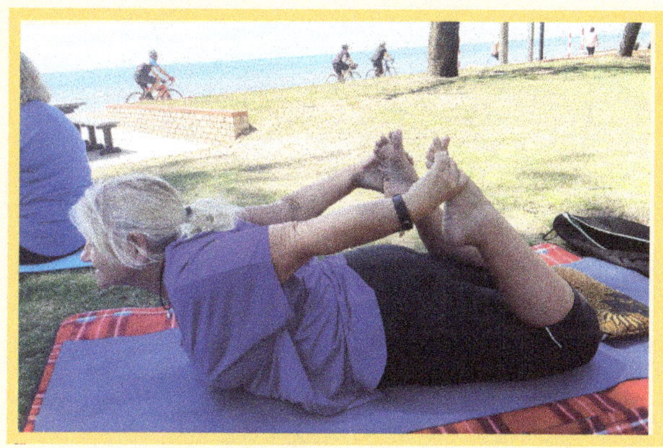

Bow pose is a strong posture that opens the chest, and the front of the body, while strengthening every muscle in the back. This pose will improve your posture and spine flexibility.

Begin with option one by lying prone with your chin on the mat, and your hands by your sides. As you breathe out, take one foot to hand and press foot towards glute for up to one minute. Change sides.
In the second round, stay with option one, or move to option two by taking both feet into hands. Breathe in, keep knees hip-distance apart and as you breathe out lift your feet up toward the sky, lifting thighs off the earth. Allow your head and chest to rise. Breathe.
Hold for up to one minute.

Release gently and move into *Child's* or *Wild Legged Child's pose.*

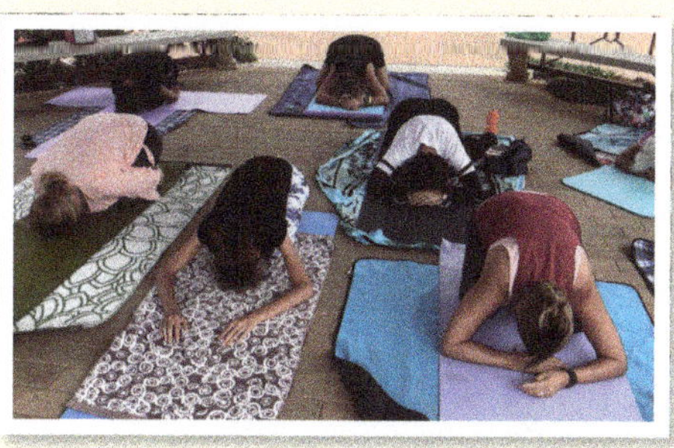

**Every day is an opportunity to love you and
accept where you are right now.**

appreciation

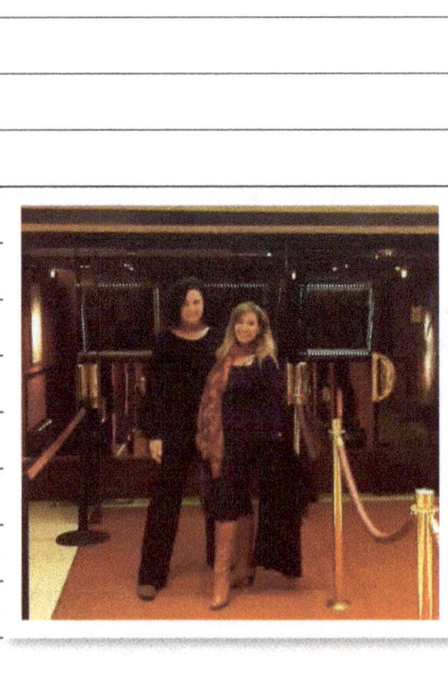

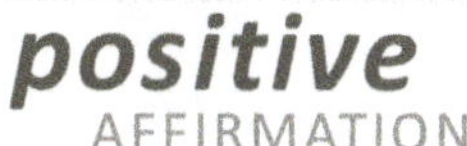

positive
AFFIRMATION

I give myself permission to shine

wisdom

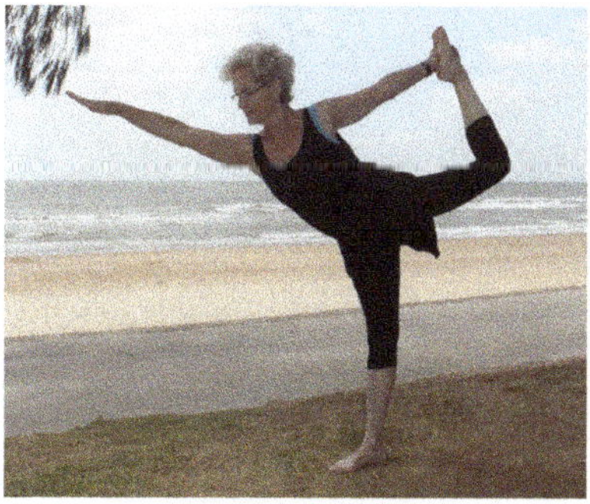

positive
AFFIRMATION

I take the very best that life has to offer

visionary

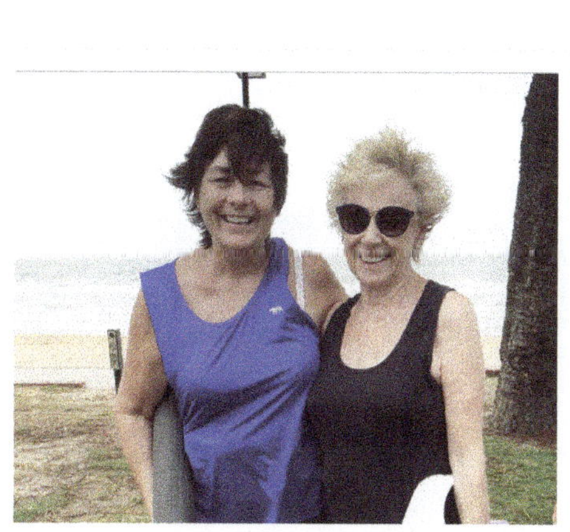

positive
AFFIRMATION

I am strong

inspirational

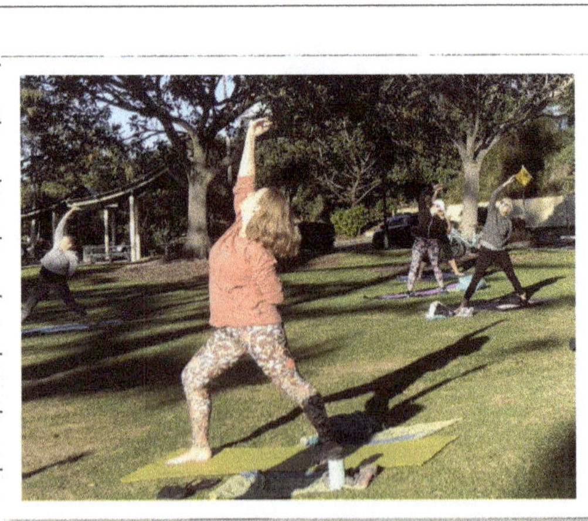

positive
AFFIRMATION

I respect myself completely

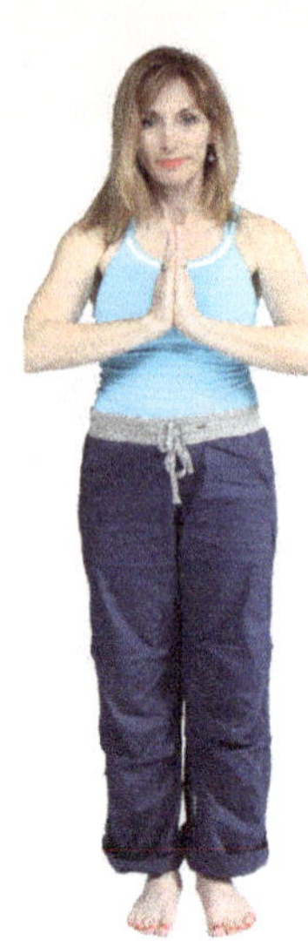

MOUNTAIN POSE

Our standing posture

Feet together or slightly apart, soft knees, tuck tailbone down, lift up pelvic floor, tummy in, lengthen spine, heart forward, press shoulders back and down, arms by side. Imagine there is a golden cord running through your spine, and feel it lifting. Lift the back of neck and notice chin tucks down. Breathe into whole lungs, including tummy and the side of ribs.

WARRIOR TWO

Opens hips and strengthens legs and core

Take a large step to the side and turn one foot to the side and the other to the front. Breathe in and open arms. Breathe out and bend leading leg. Straighten the back leg and press the outer edge of foot onto the mat. If knees are uncomfortable, adjust feet until knees are comfortable. Press knee out to open hip. Open hips to the front by pressing the top hip back and the lower sitting bone forward. As you get stronger, you will be able to deepen the bend in your leg towards a ninety degree angle.

After *Warrior Two*, release for *Side Lunge.*

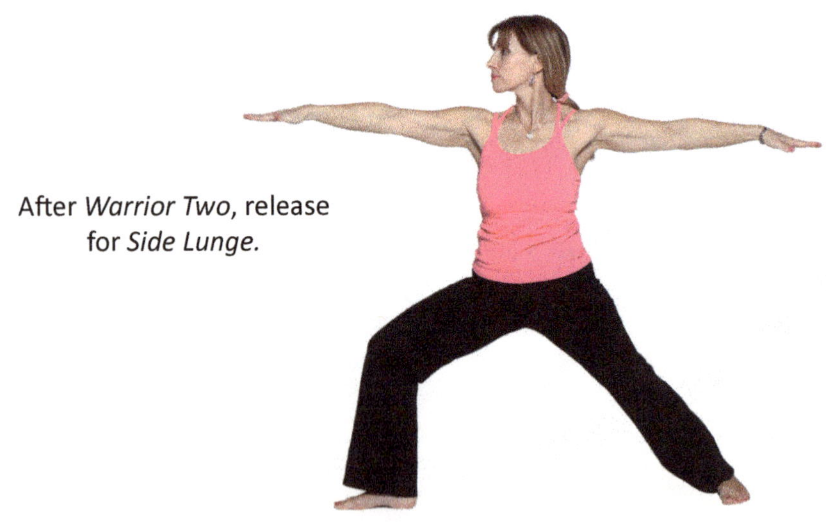

SIDE LUNGE

Opens hips, lengthens spine, waist, ankles and thighs

Option 1: Inhale deeply and on the exhale, reach over the side, resting lower arm on thigh and stretch top arm either straight up or overhead, rotate the shoulder back and down. Press top hip back and lower sitting bone forward. Press knee out to open hip.

Option 2: Lower arm towards the earth.

Option 3: Top arm bends and slides down your back. Press lower arm down until shoulder and knee are level, take arm under leg as though you are going to grab your butt with your hand, but take hold of your other hand instead in a monkey grip. Press the top shoulder back and look up at the sky.

Breathe and hold for several breaths. Release, rise, roll shoulders forward and back. Change sides. Turn feet out for *Victory Pose.*

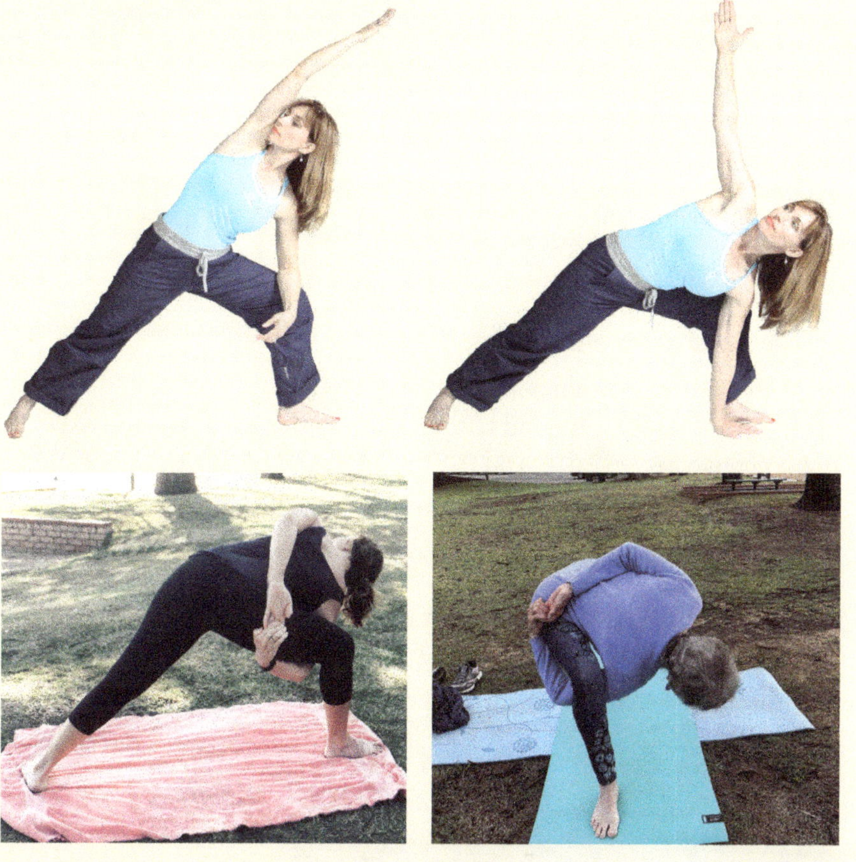

BREATHE

LOVE

PEACE

PERFECT
HEALTH

PROSPERITY

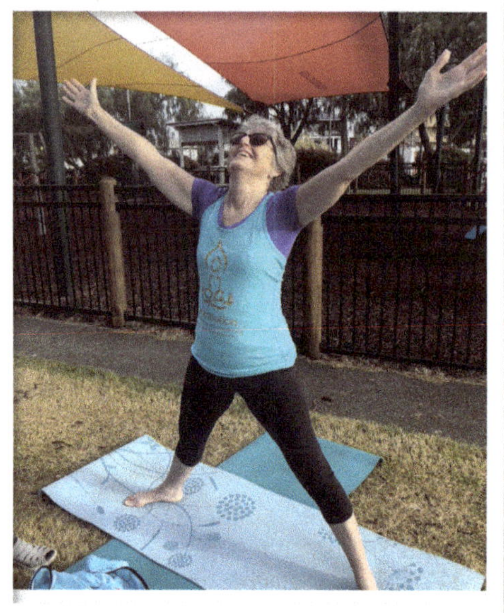

Step out and open arms, legs, feet and mind. Lift heart and look up. You are in the posture of success. Visualise your success whatever that means for you. Breathe. Expand. Visualise the perfect scene. You can do this. You are doing this. never give up because you deserve to succeed at your goals.

.

Wrap yourself in love and release your arms.
Take the hands behind the back to prepare for Forward Fold.

In Yoga, each pose is as individual

as you are and how you express each pose

will be unique to you.

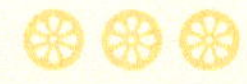

FORWARD FOLD
WITH ARMS OVERHEAD

Clasp hands behind back, stretch arms, fold forward and raise arms over head. Keep knees soft. If there is any pain in your back, bend knees. At first you may not move very far. Be patient, this is where you are right now, and that's ok.

Hold this pose for up to one minute, inhale, bend knees, lift head and with a straight back rise, release hands and exhale. It's important to rise slowly so that your blood pressure has a chance to stabilise. If you come up too quickly, you might feel dizzy.

Repeat the entire sequence on the other side.

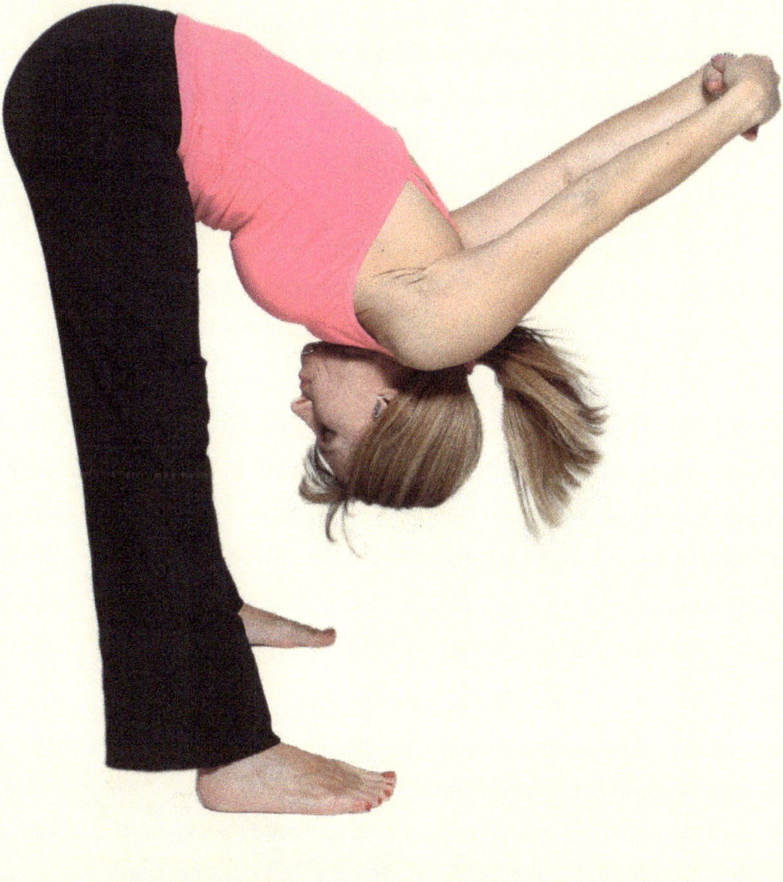

BEND AND STRETCH

From *Forward Fold*, bend the knees and softly rise, taking arms over head and hands to heart. From here we *Bend and Stretch*

Option one, if you have high blood pressure or for any reason you'd prefer not to bend forward, bend and stretch from standing.

Bend the knees, keep pressing the knees open as you press heels to earth. Eyes straight ahead. Bend to your capacity, then straighten. Repeat for up to 10 rounds. Breathing in as you rise, out as you bend.

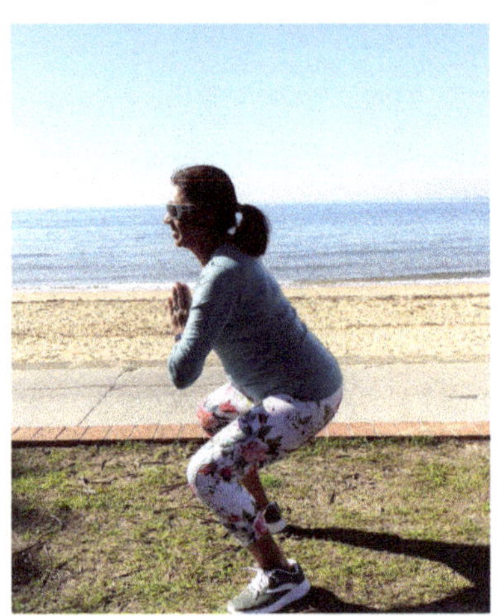
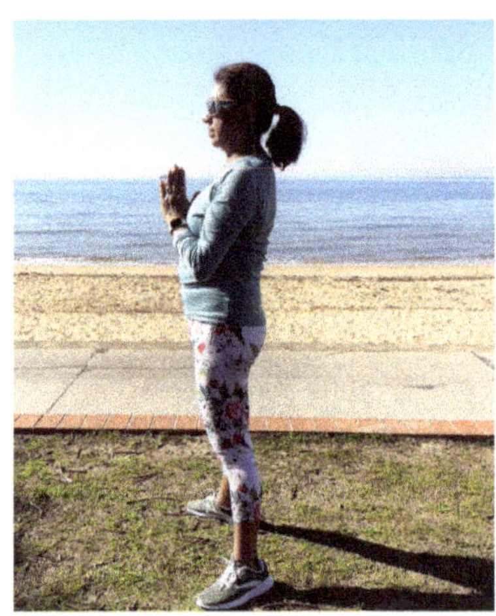

Option two keep your hands on the earth
and bend and stretch from there.

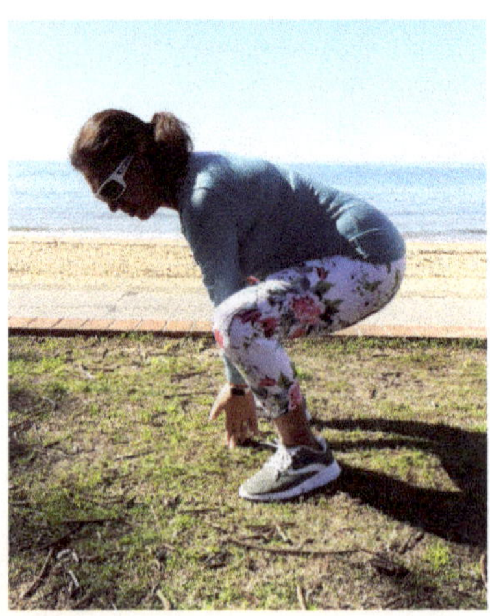
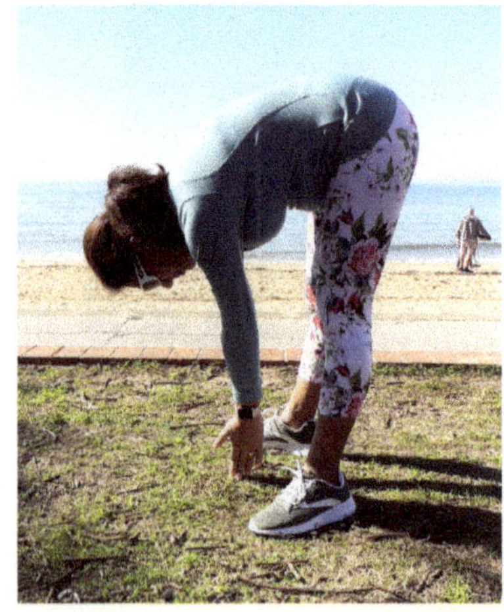

Option three; *Hindi Squat* to *Forward Fold*. Keep the elbows pressing knees open. Breathe in to *Hindi* and out to *Forward Fold*.

Finish in the bend. Rise to release and let go.

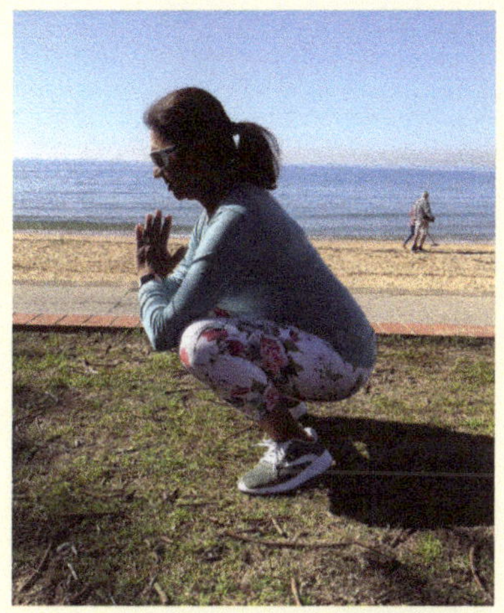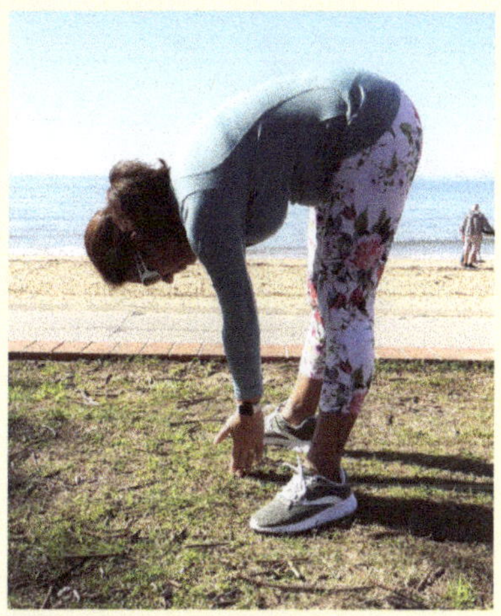

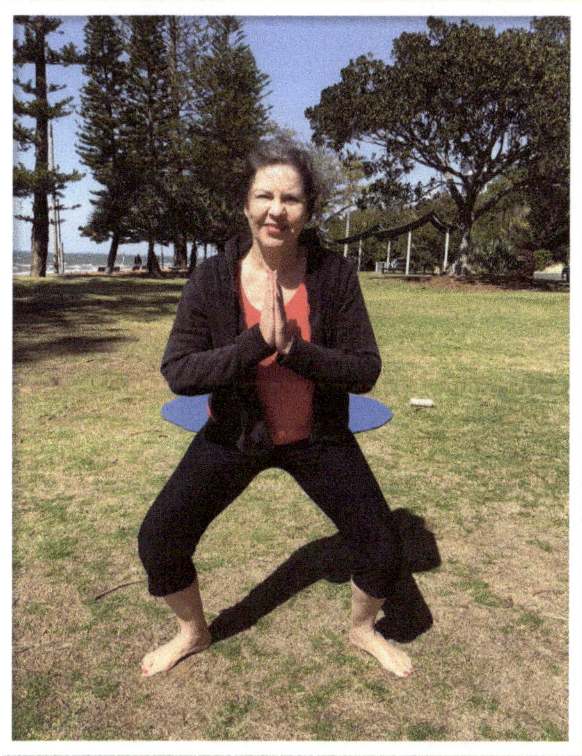

meditation

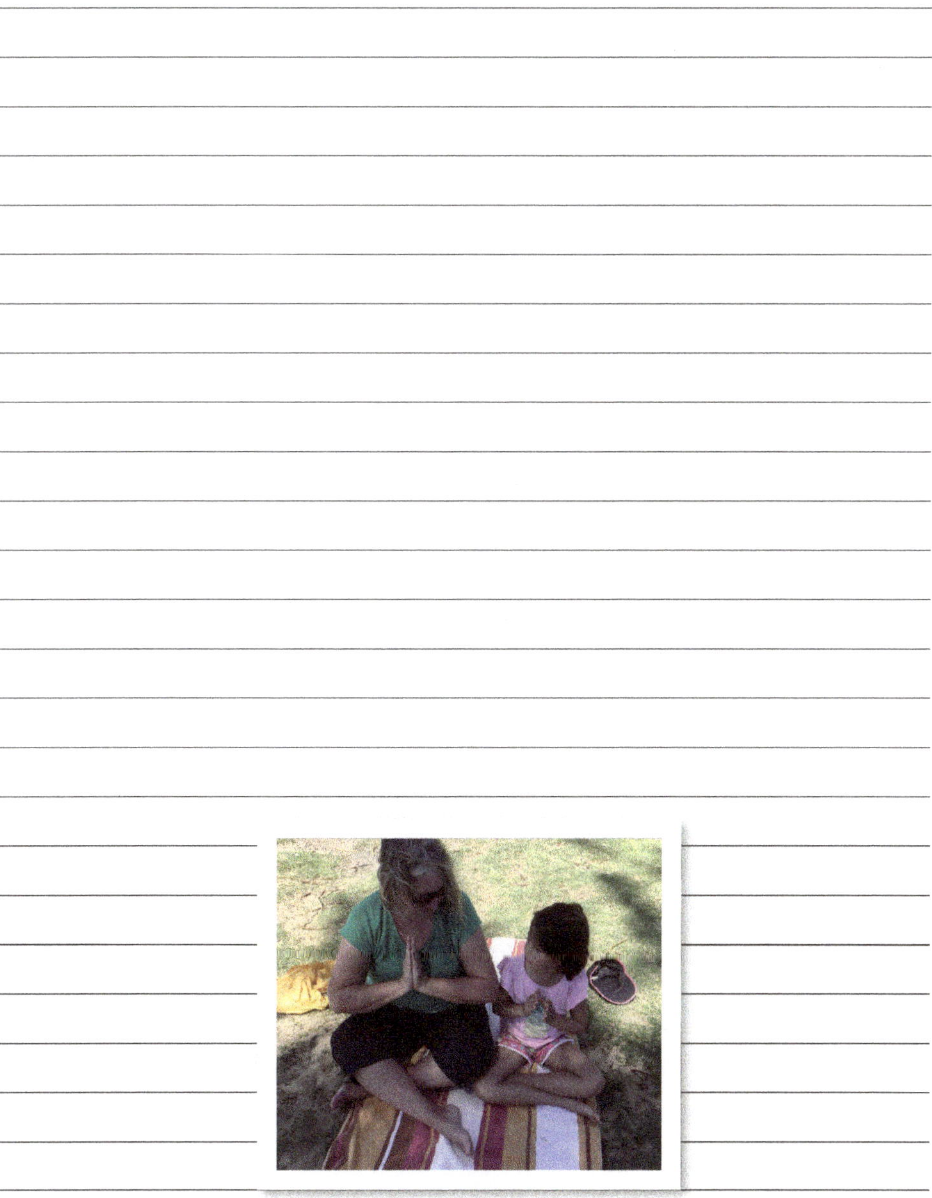

positive
AFFIRMATION

I am focused on my dreams

focus

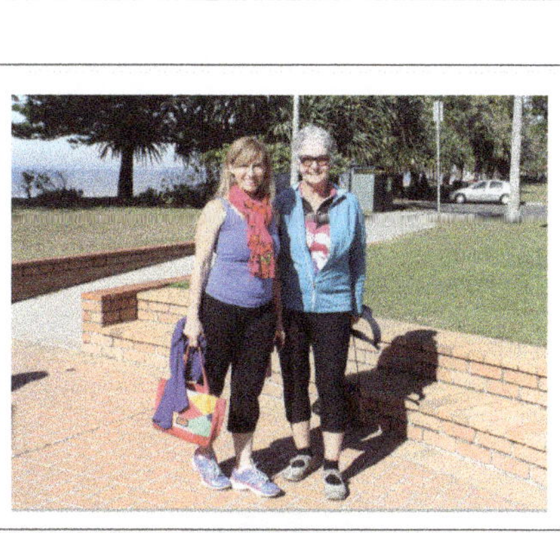

positive
AFFIRMATION

I am loving and kind to myself and my family

considerate

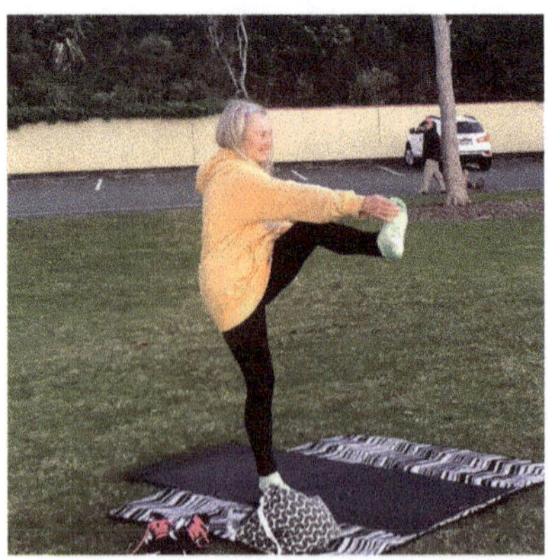

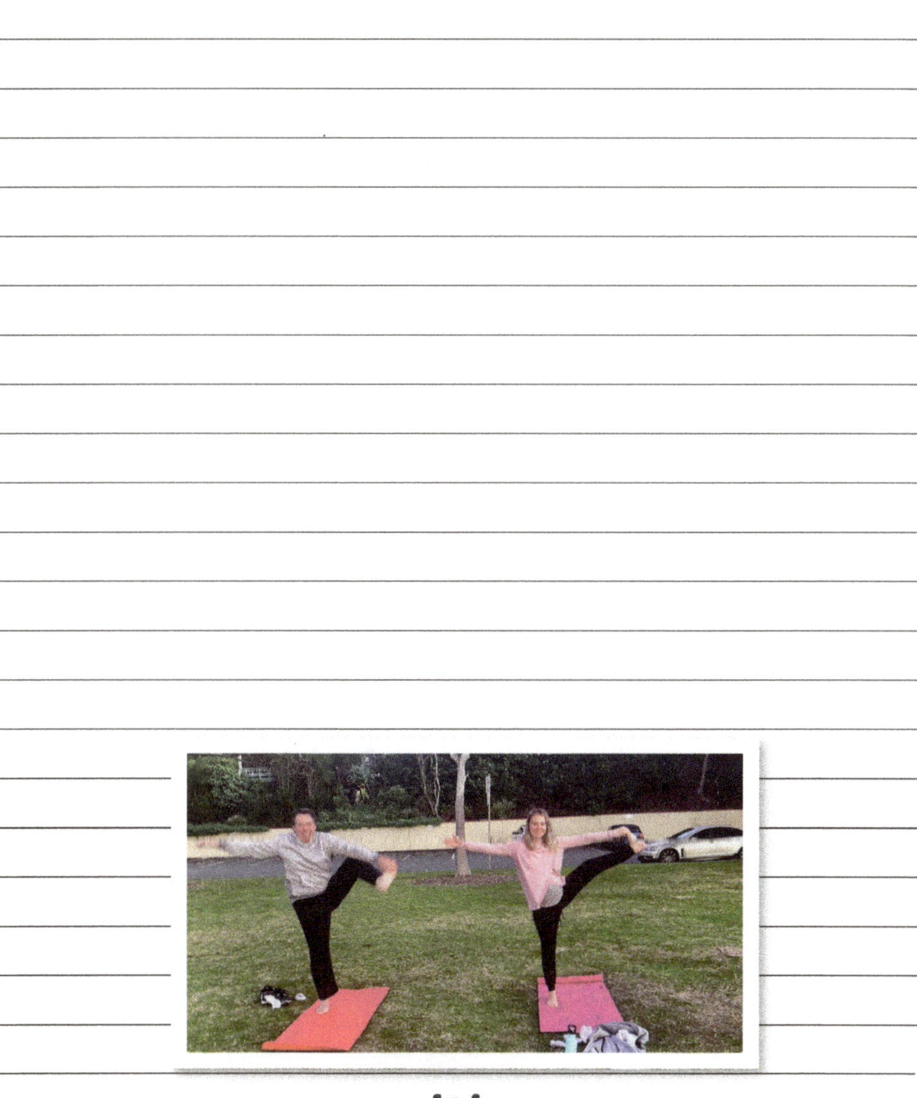

positive
AFFIRMATION

I choose my own destiny

balance

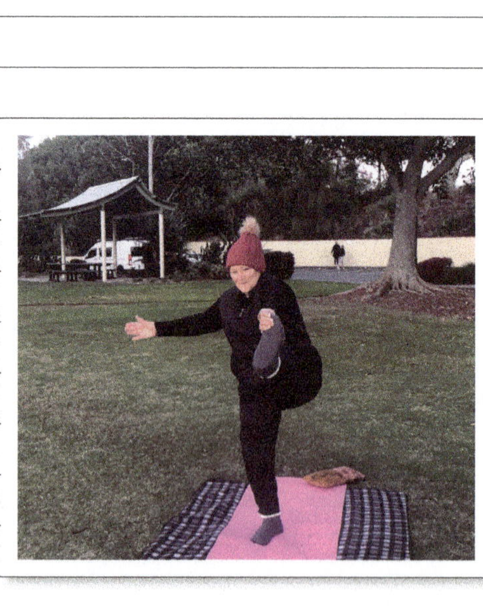

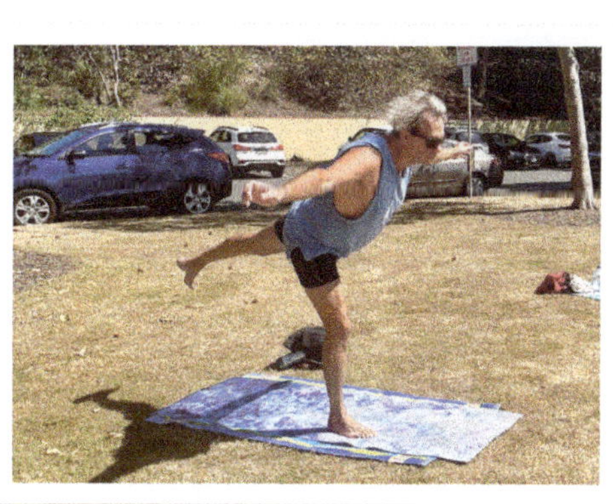

positive
AFFIRMATION

I am gentle with myself

Balance

Yoga helps us balance life because life, like balance, requires focus, mindfulness and the letting go of 'shoulds'.

When you balance your body you balance your mind. When life is in balance you work when you need to, rest when you need to, and love yourself all the time.

Follow your heart to lead yourself into the perfect balance for you.

Notice what you say to yourself during a yoga balance. Your self-talk will indicate how you manage your focus. When balance in yoga is achieved, life balance improves.

Just like life; staying present helps you focus on the task at hand, and being distracted can cause you to lose your balance.

If you are stressed, keep yourself attuned to your breath so you can hear your intuition guiding you towards a better outcome.

Balance postures grow neuroplasticity. This means as you balance, you are developing brain cells. These cells will not only help you improve balance, but increase your ability to solve problems and respond to events. For instance, when an elderly person falls over, it isn't always because they are weaker, but because their brains are slower at processing the information to correct the balance. Neuroplasticity helps the brain process faster. Yoga helps the elderly stay in their own home longer.

Yoga can be practised at all ages as there are options for everyone.

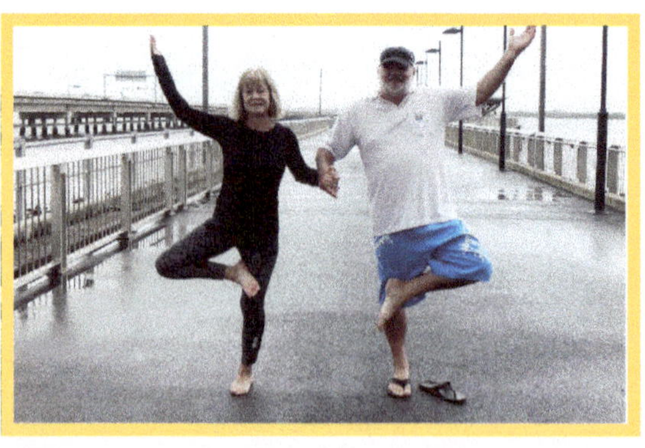

TREE POSE

Begin in Mountain pose. From Mountain pose, feel your balance and shift weight to one foot. Tuck other heel in front of ankle for option one, foot below knee for option two, and above knee for option three, arms to sky, pressing palms together. Hold and breathe for up to thirty seconds. Stay centred—tummy in, tailbone down, heart forward, shoulders back. Hands in prayer, breathe in and stretch.

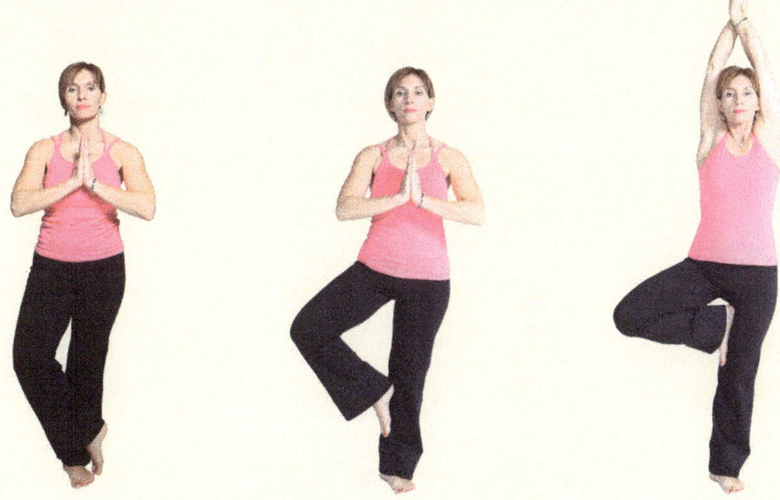

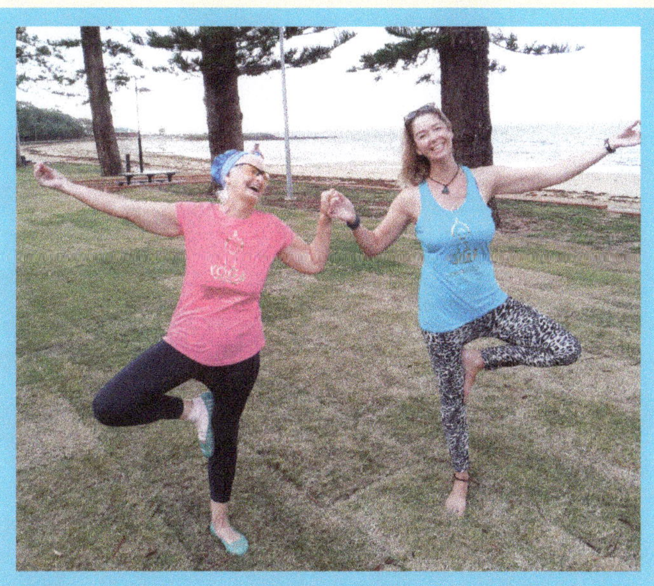

Balance
EAGLE POSE

Shoulder and hip flexibility. Balance and Focus

From Mountain. Breathe in and take arms out, then swoop right arm under and bring top arm to the crook of lower arm, wrap the lower palm into the upper palm and press. For a softer option, take arm across or bring forearms together. Breathe in and lift right leg up and cross over your left leg. Wrap foot around calf, sink into a deeper bend. Square the hips and shoulders. Press palms forward. Breathe. Softer options are to balance right toe on the earth.

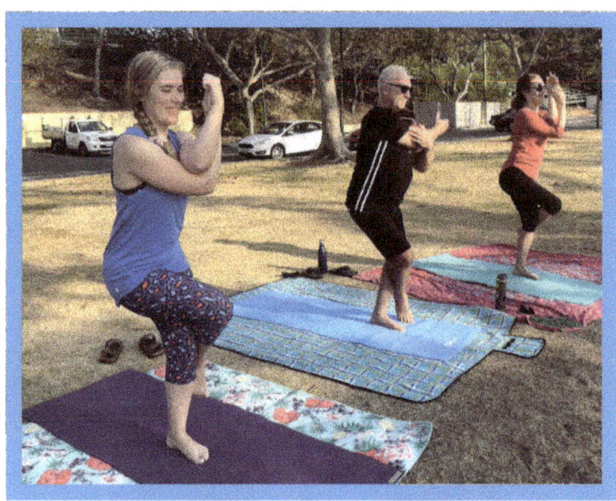

AEROPLANE
Strong and balanced

From Mountain pose. Step one foot forward, lift the arms high. Place weight onto the front foot and slowly lift the back foot,
stretch arms out to the side, like the wings of a plane.

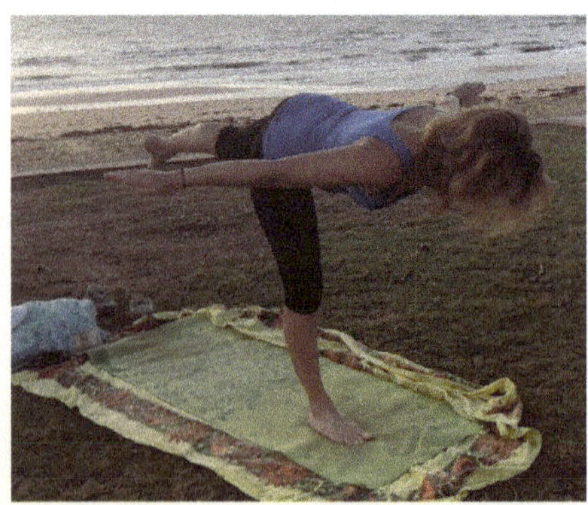

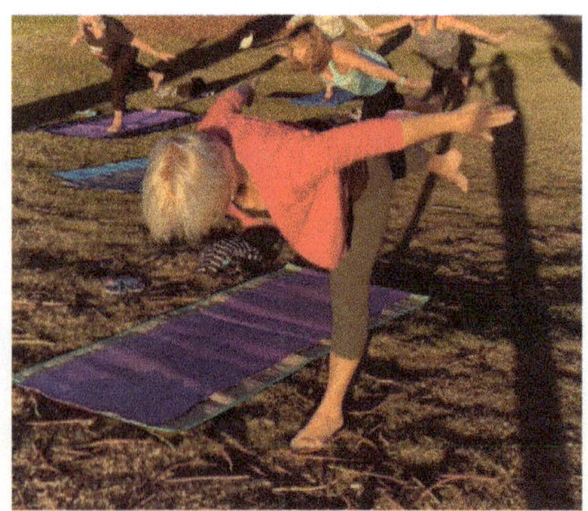

BIRD POSE

From Hindi squat, place your hands on the earth, rise to your toes,
lean forward and place shins on upper arms. Keep your butt down
(like a crouch) and lean on your hands to take your weight.
Slowly lift one foot, then the other. Take your time. This is a strong pose.

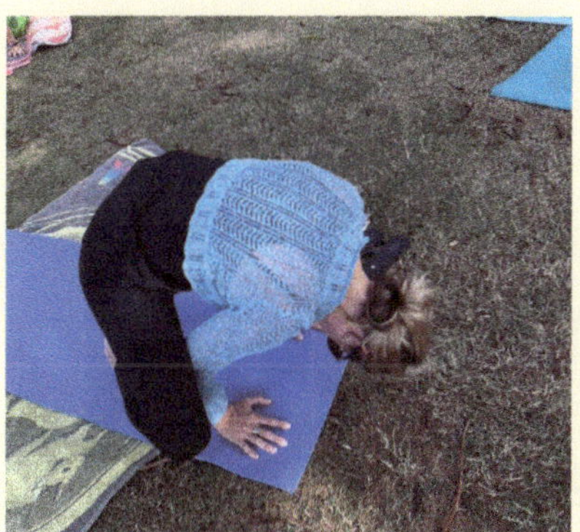
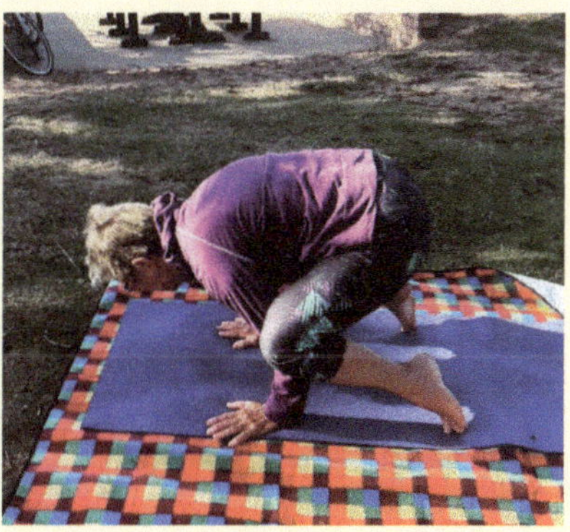

Just for FUN

DOWN DOG DOWN DOG DOWN DOG

The girls had fun one Monday morning seeing if they could make a
Downward Dog Daisy chain.
I think they did a marvellous job.

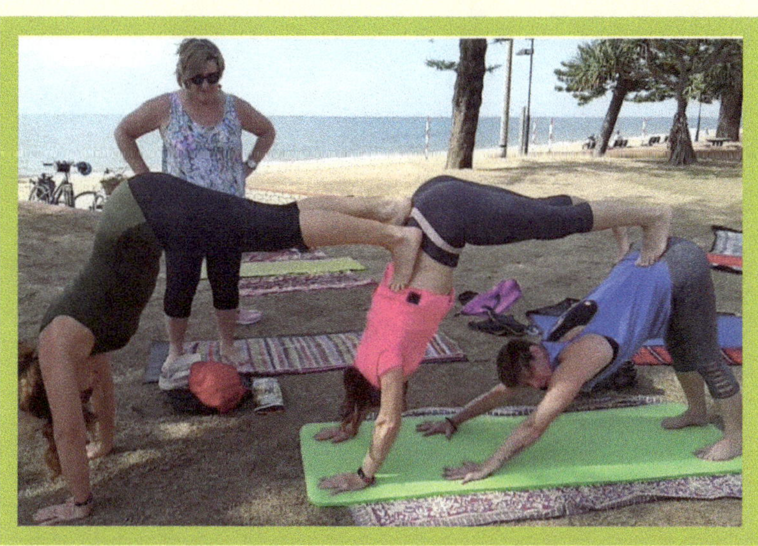

HAND TO TOE POSE TO THE SIDE

Hand to Toe pose can take leg out to the side or to the front.
Begin in *Mountain pose*, breathe in and slowly bring knee to chest and hold
with your hands. Stay here for option one. Option two, take hand onto inside of
leg to slide hand to foot. Slowly stretch leg out to side.

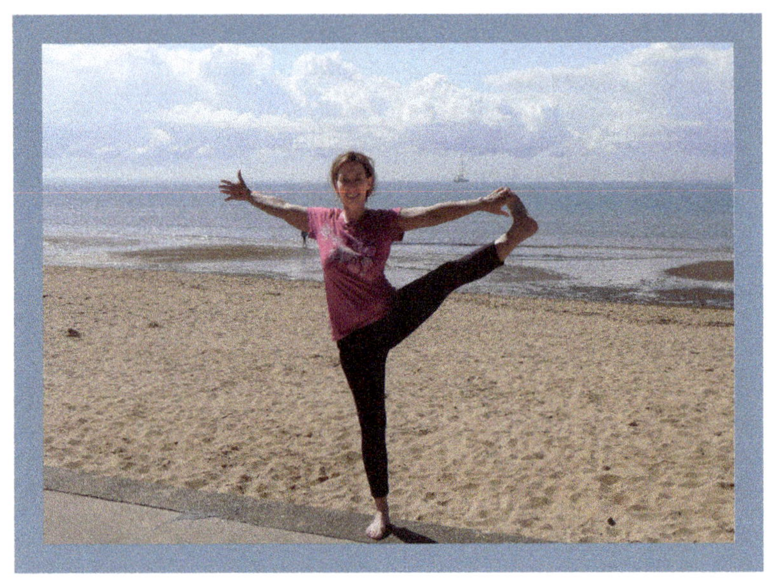

HAND TO TOE POSE TO THE FRONT

From *Mountain pose* lift knee to chest, place hands on foot, and slowly stretch leg out to the front. You can keep both hands on foot, straightening spine and legs, or you can place one hand to foot and release the other hand to the side.

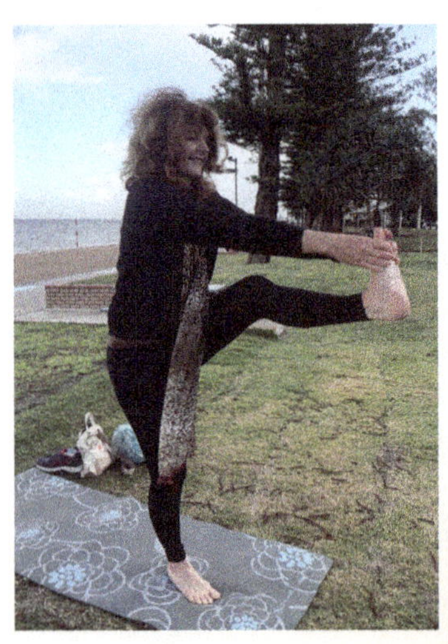

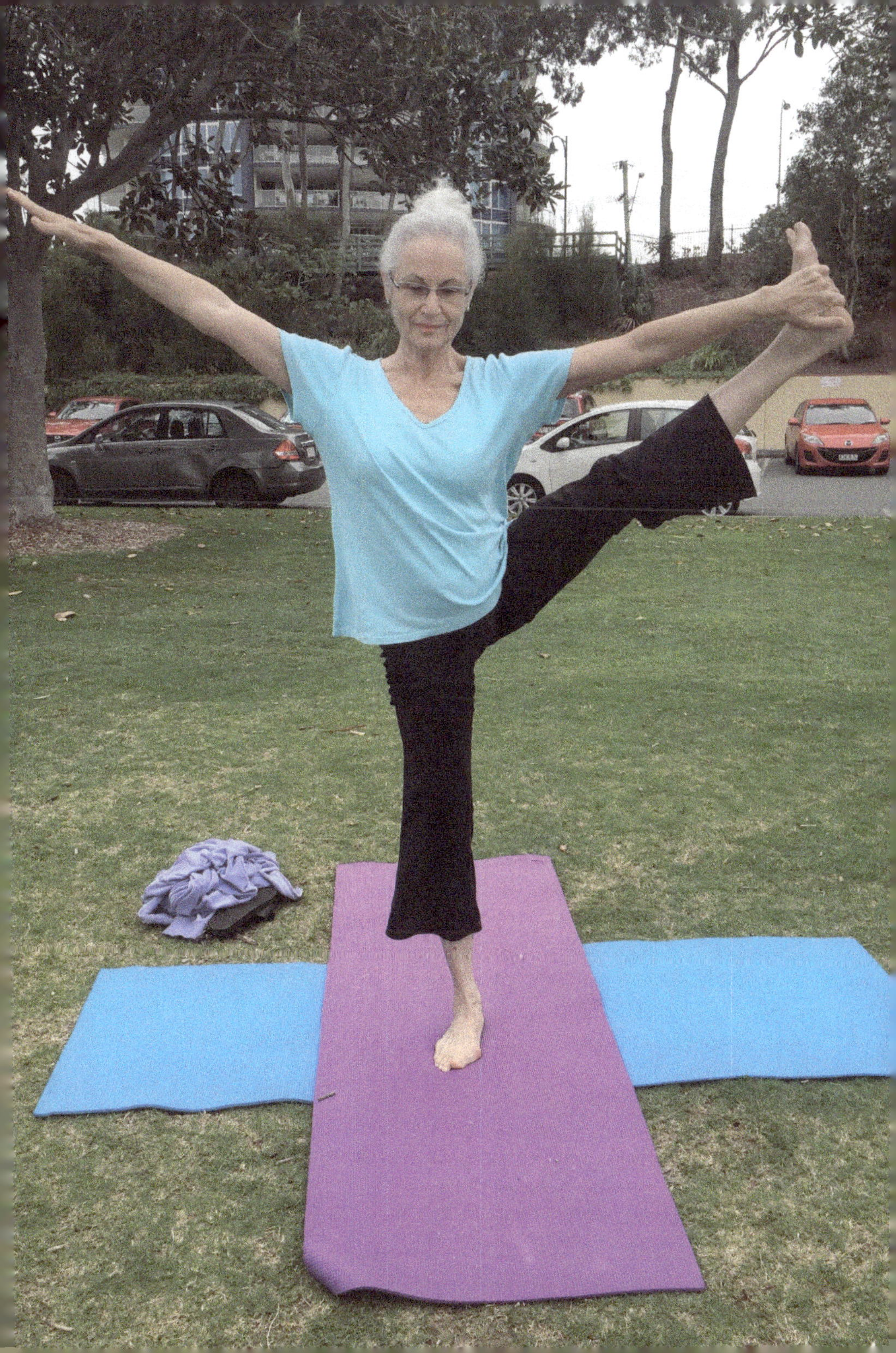

dedication

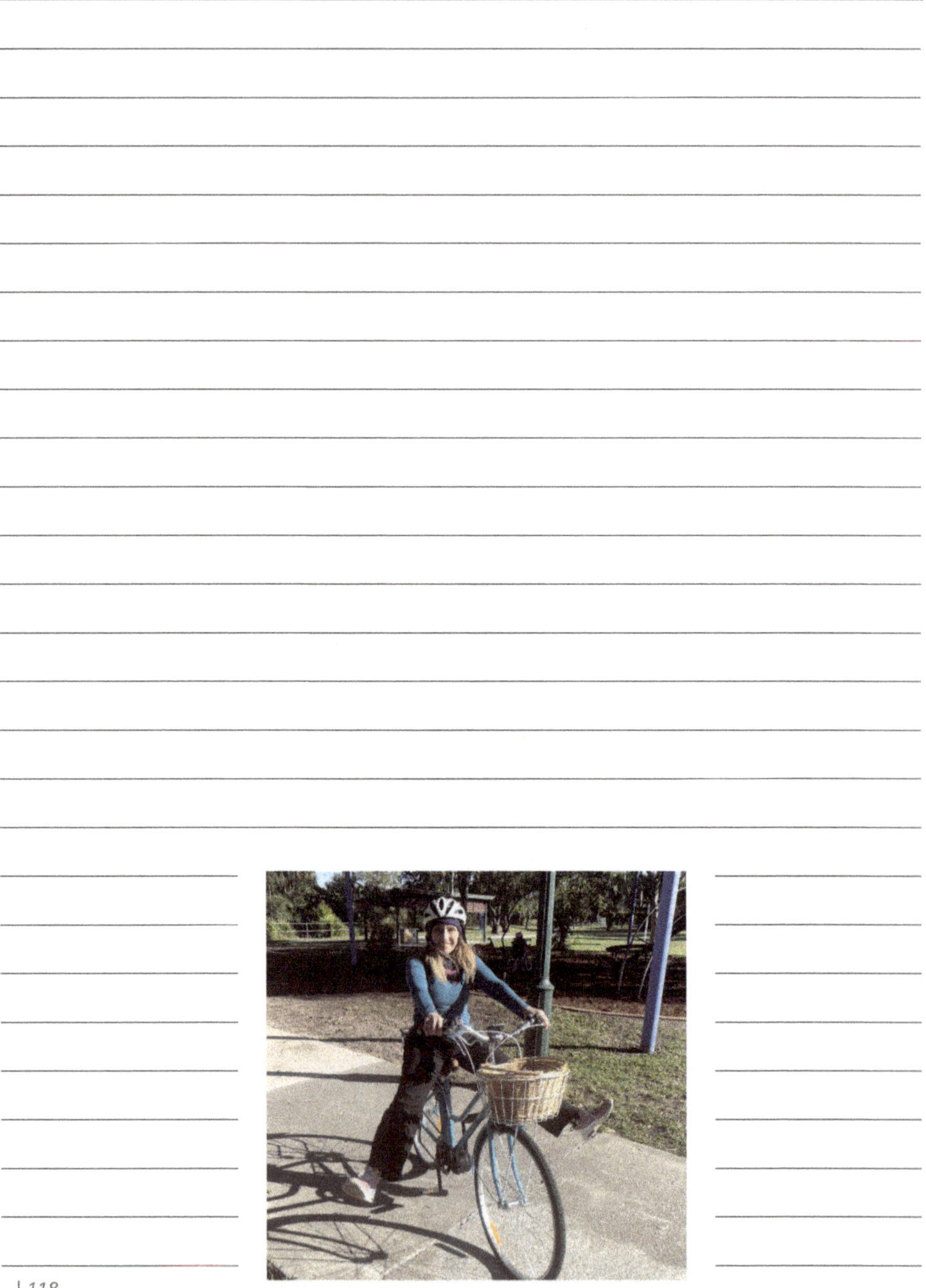

dedication

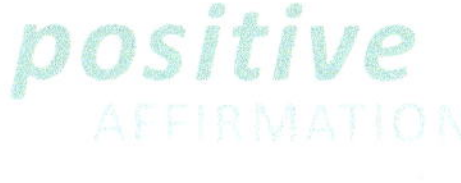
positive
AFFIRMATION
connection is key

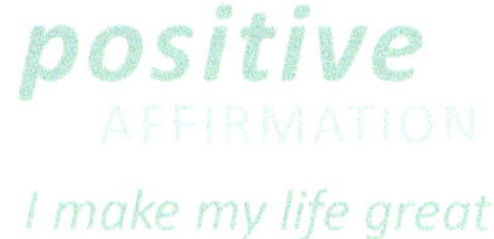

positive
AFFIRMATION
I make my life great

free

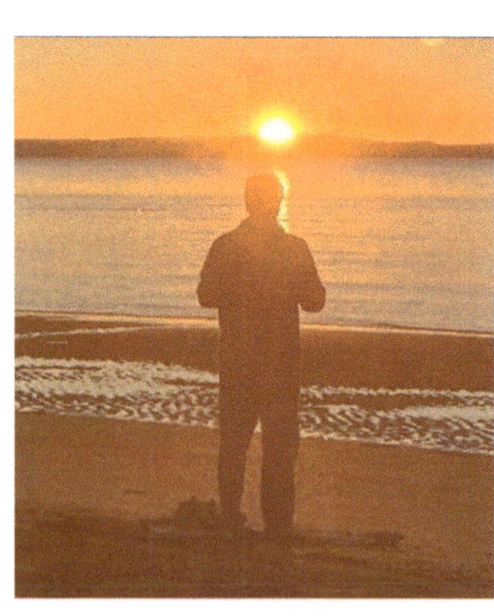

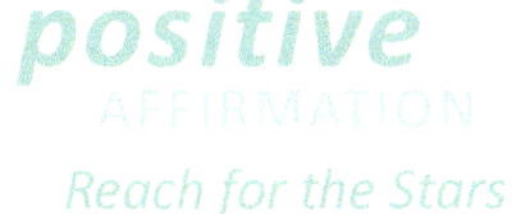

Dancer's Pose

Grace and empowerment

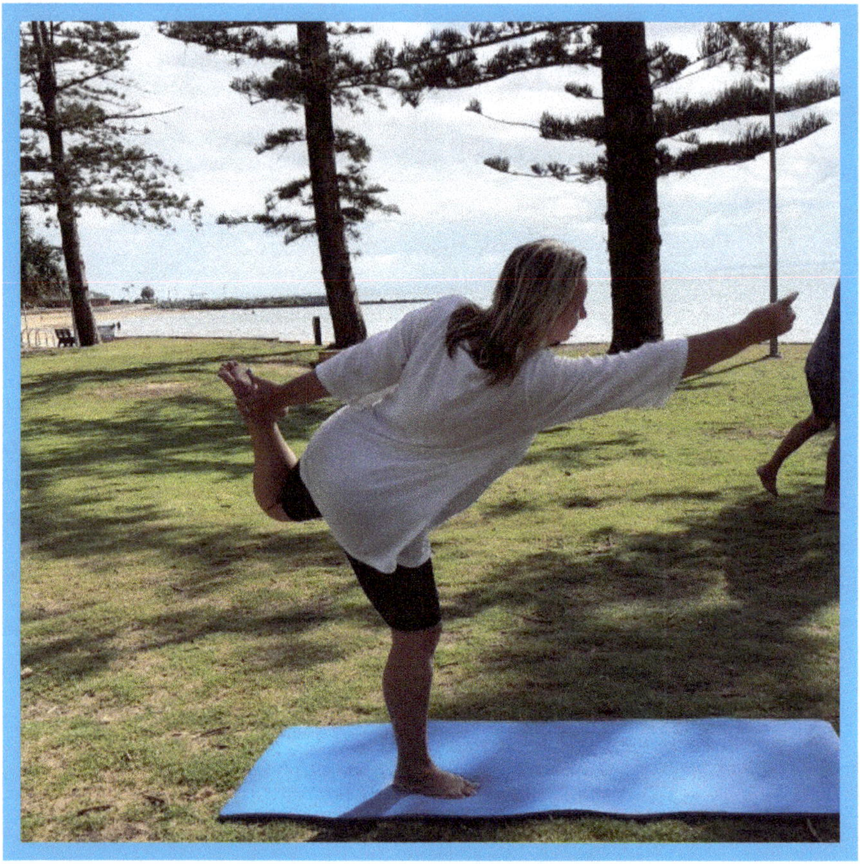

From *Mountain pose*, step right foot forward and take your weight onto the front foot. Back foot can stay close to the earth for option one.

For option two, take your back foot into your hand. Breathe in, and as you breathe out press body towards the earth as you press and lift back hand and foot to sky for *Dancer's pose*. Lift heart and front hand. Stay focused and hold for up to thirty seconds. Release to a forward fold, bend and rock your body to release. Change sides.

Trust yourself

You know yourself better than anyone

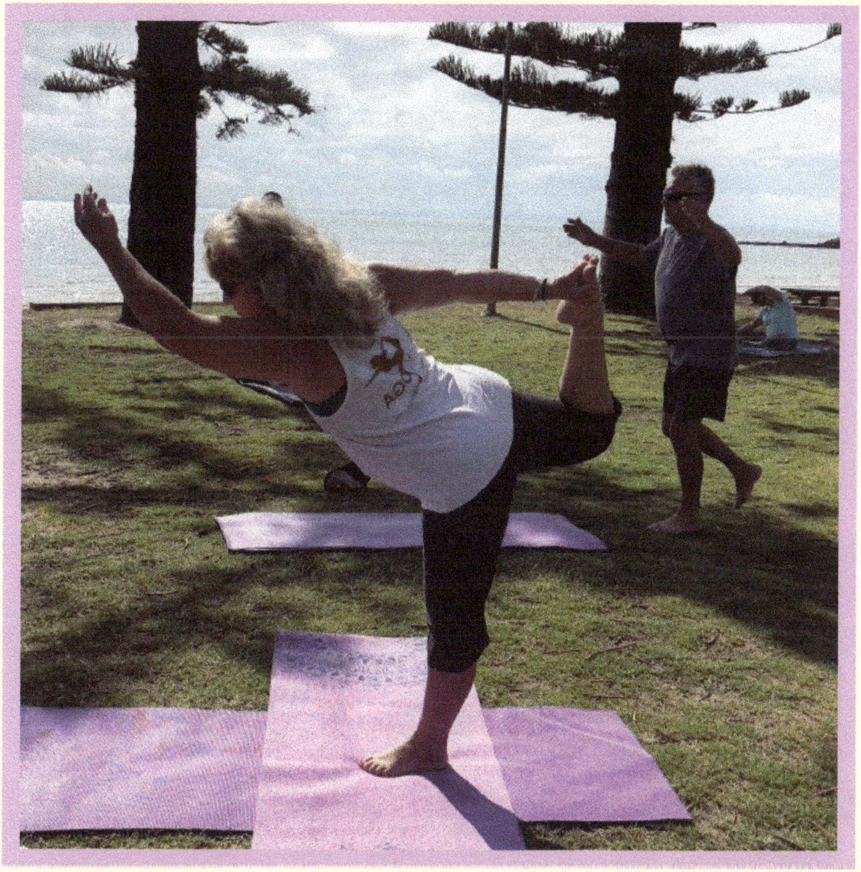

You are already perfect, just as you are

Breathe   Balance   Focus   Believe

JABIRU

Begin in *Mountain pose*, breathe arms above head and bring hands to heart. Lean on right leg, and place left foot across with toe resting on the earth for option one; take foot across knee for option two; or place foot high on thigh in half lotus for option three. Hold for up to one minute and release. Take a few breaths and change sides.

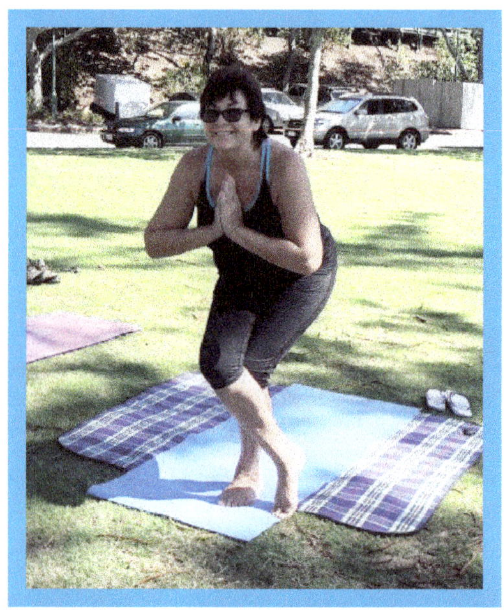

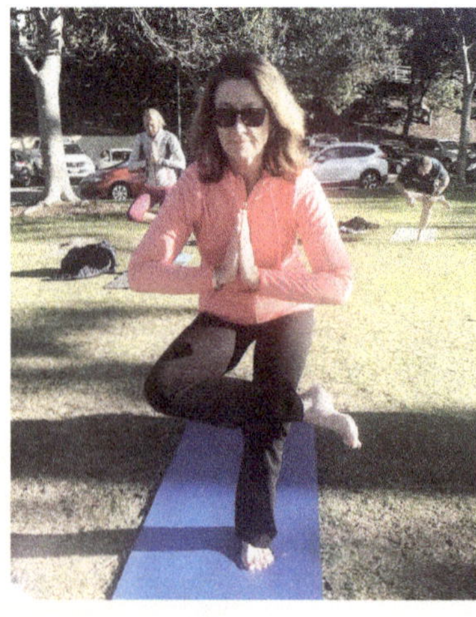

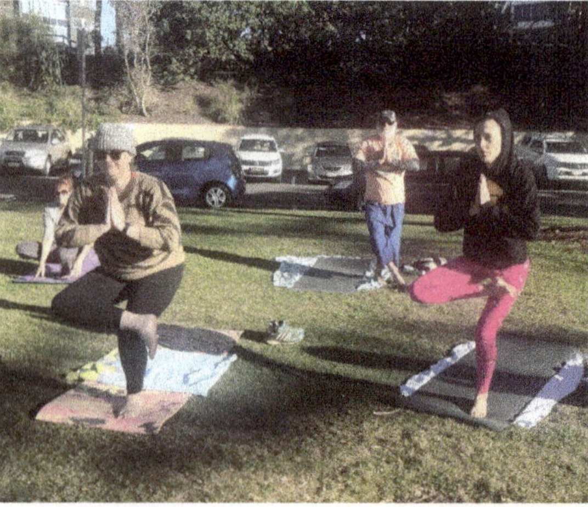

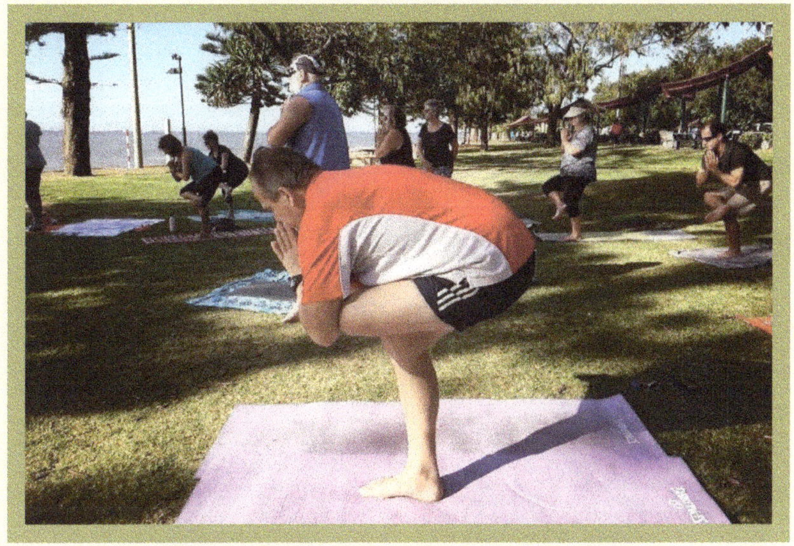

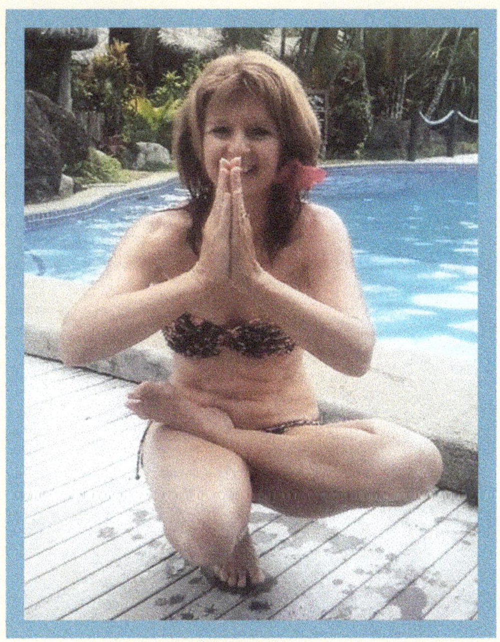

If you are in option three, you can extend this posture by deepening your squat, place your hands onto the earth to take your weight, and then crouch with your foot still resting on the supporting thigh. Take your hands to your side to find your balance, then place your hands back to your heart. When you release this posture, come up the reverse of how you went down.

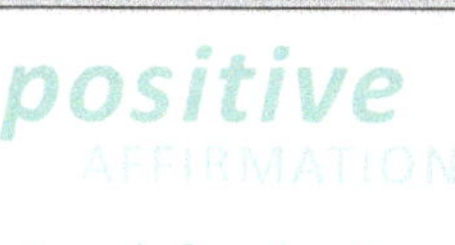

Reach for the Stars

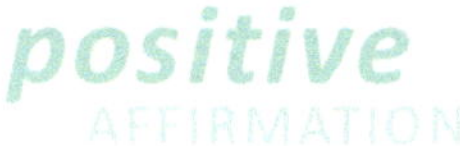

Mindfulness helps me stay focused, balanced and happy

optimistic

positive
AFFIRMATION

Our love can change the world

positive
AFFIRMATION

Strong, beautiful, balanced and flexible

Loving yourself

Accepting yourself just as you are is the relief your mind and body is looking for. Let go of where you 'should be' and accept where you are. From here, you move forward with ease.

Surround yourself with positive people, think positive thoughts and watch as life raises you towards your greatest dreams and ultimate desires.

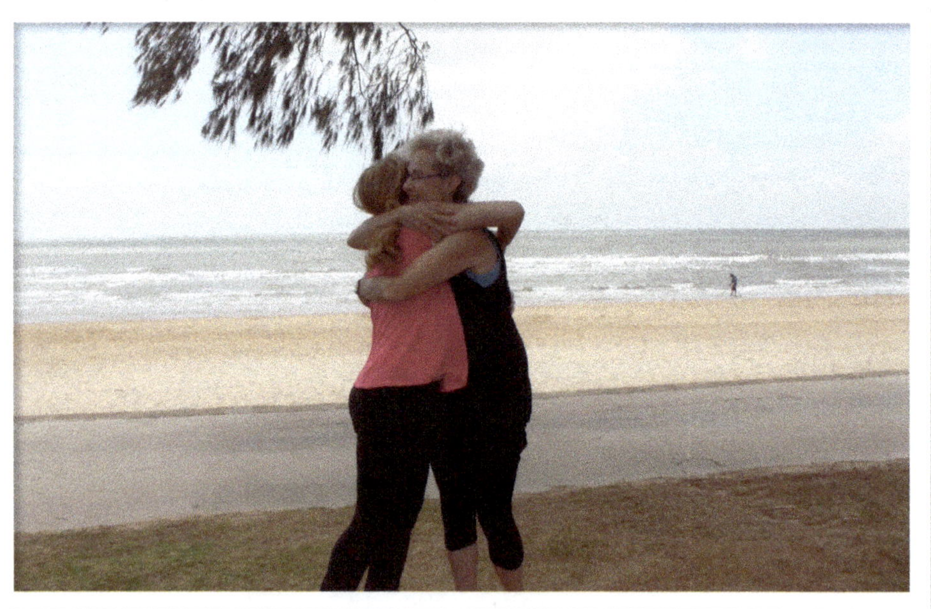

In the end what will matter to you most is;
How well did I love?

How well did I live?
How well did I learn to let go?

Carl Jung

FRIENDSHIPS

Friendships are an important part of life. Friends help us connect with our community and helps us feel like we belong.
Making friends can be hard for some people. Friendships usually form through common interests and through socialising.
When people have difficulty socialising and expressing themselves, they can find it hard to make friends.
To help people make friends and feel like a part of your community, smile and be friendly. Accept others just as they are, and be as true to yourself as you can.

Friendships help us find connection

FRIENDS

Friends help us know who we are, by their acceptance of us, and their positive reflection about who we are. A friend is someone who believes in your hopes and dreams, someone who likes and loves you, just as you are. A friend will listen to your problems without sharing them with others.
A friend is someone who makes you feel good about yourself.

Friends and community give us a sense of belonging.

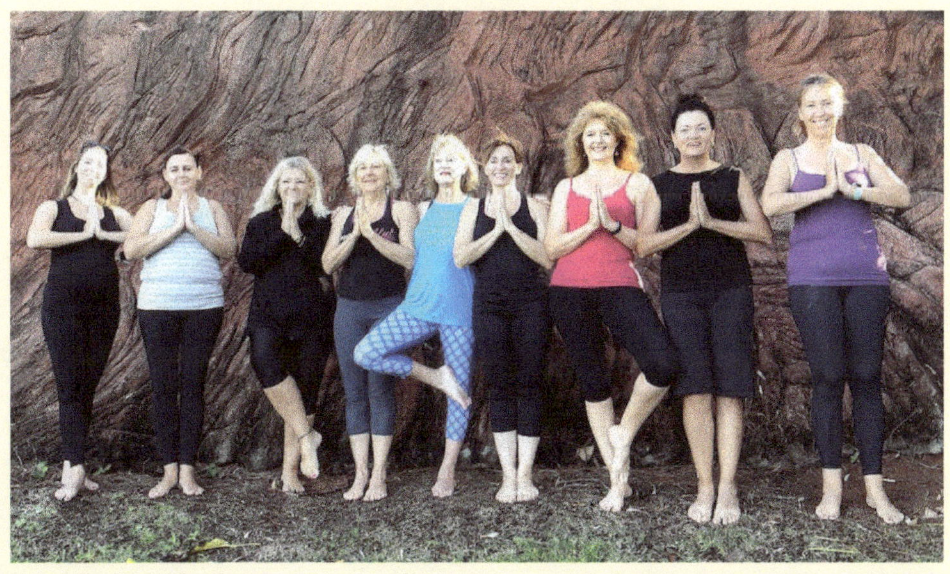

Your breath

Deep breathing is your bodies way of knowing that 'Everything is ok. All is well. I am safe.' And when your body recognises this, it responds by switching off stress and switching on peace. Deep breathing helps to strengthen the vegas nerve.

Your *vegas nerve* is the *'rest and digest* nerve.' Strengthening this nerve will build your resilience to stress, increase your capacity to find peace, and help to repair your hippocampus (the part of your brain that helps you remember). You can strengthen your vegas nerve by taking long slow breaths, and by lengthening your exhale. Gargling, singing, and humming also strengthen the vegas nerve. So next time you're in class and your practising *The Humming Bee* breath, or *AUM,* or the *Ujjay breath;* you're not only coming to peace now, but your ability to find peace in every day life will be boosted.

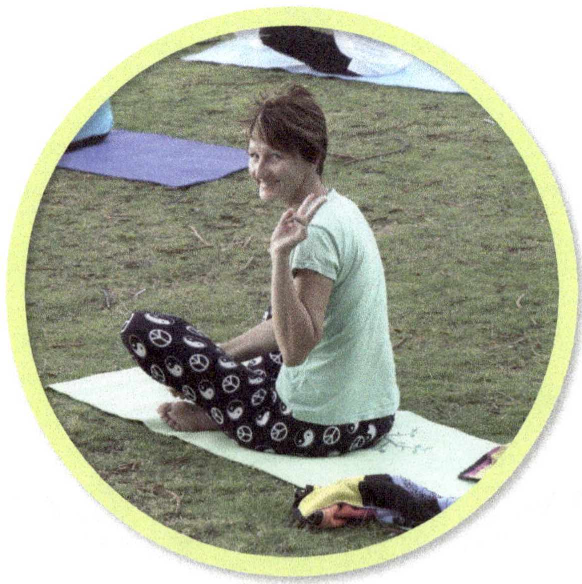

If only you knew how deeply you deserve to be loved

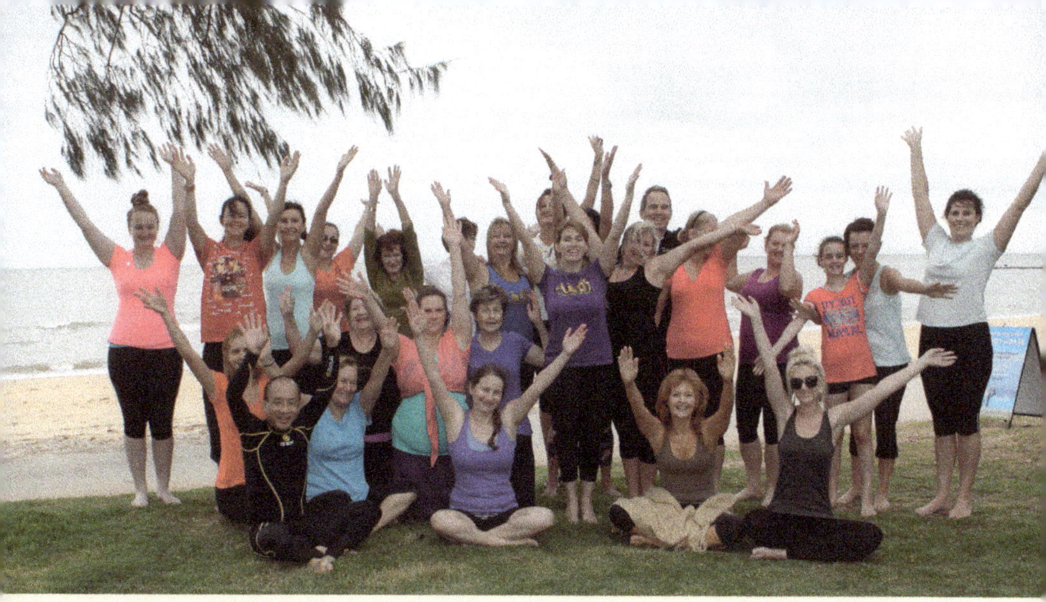

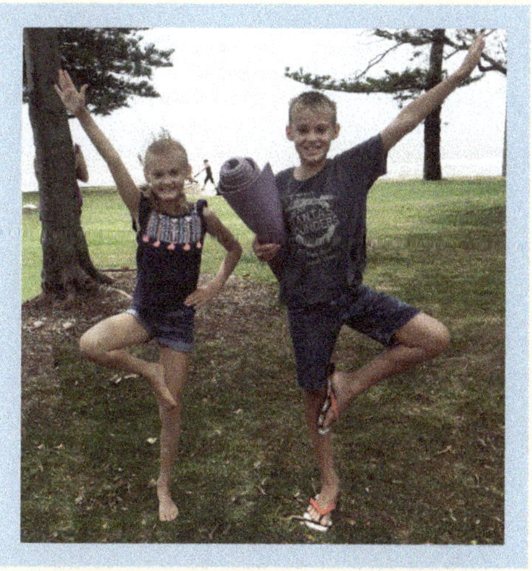

Deep breaths every hour

Throughout the day, take three deep breaths every hour, relax your shoulders and visualise something peaceful and happy.

This will train your mind and body to move towards peace and away from stress. It sounds easy doesn't it? It will take you less than one minute and will radically change your day.

BREATHE   BALANCE   BELIEVE

confidence

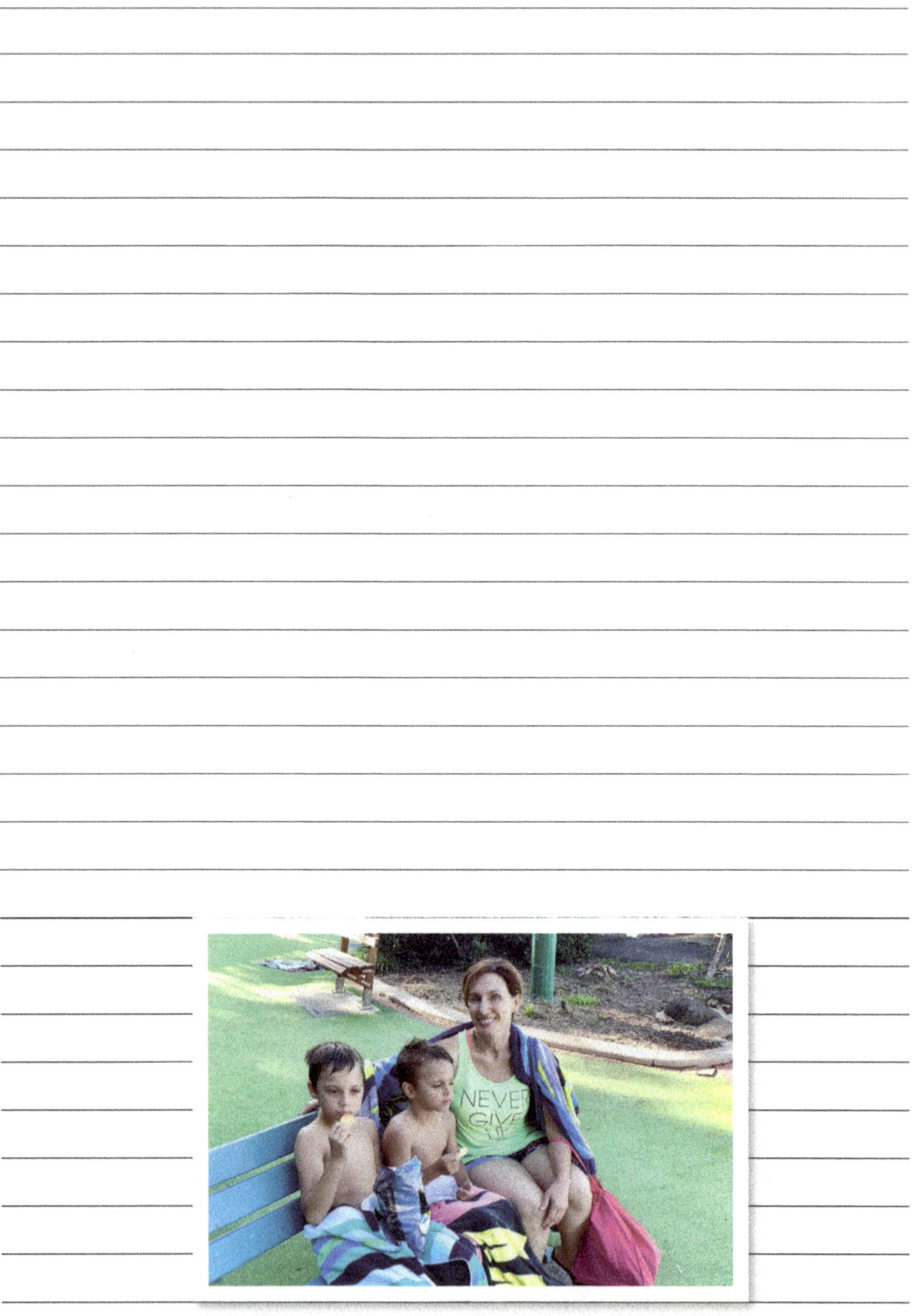

positive
AFFIRMATION

I follow my joy and happiness to where I want to go

inspired

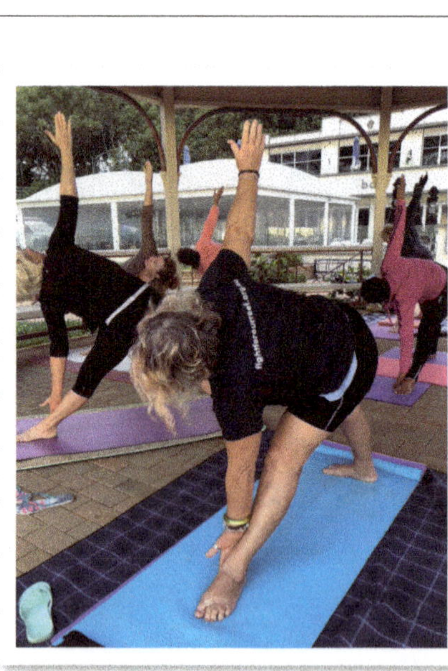

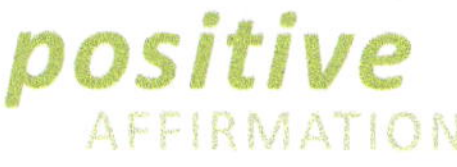

positive
AFFIRMATION
I follow my path

winner

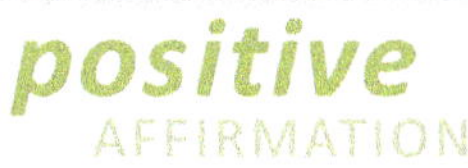

I honour my journey

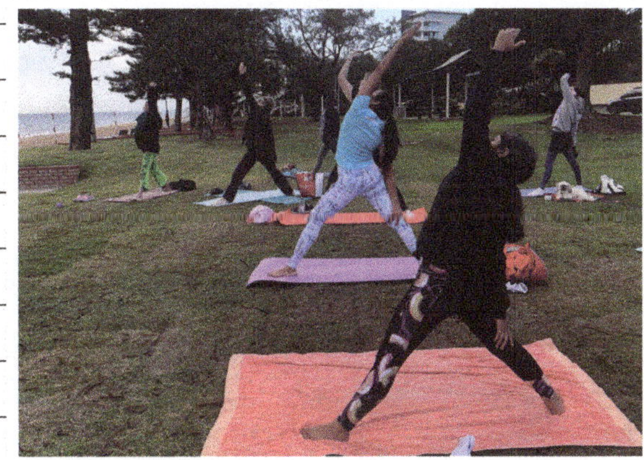

positive
AFFIRMATION
I relax and breathe

A Rhythmic Pattern

Use your breath to move from one posture to the next. Respect your body and go at the pace that is perfect for you. Soften as you need to.

DOWNWARD DOG

Releases shoulders and hamstrings.

Slide hands forward at shoulder width apart. Press heels towards the earth and lift tailbone towards the sky. Tuck toes in and rise to *Downward Facing Dog*. Separate shoulders by rotating shoulders out and elbows in. Remain in *Downward Dog* for several breaths.

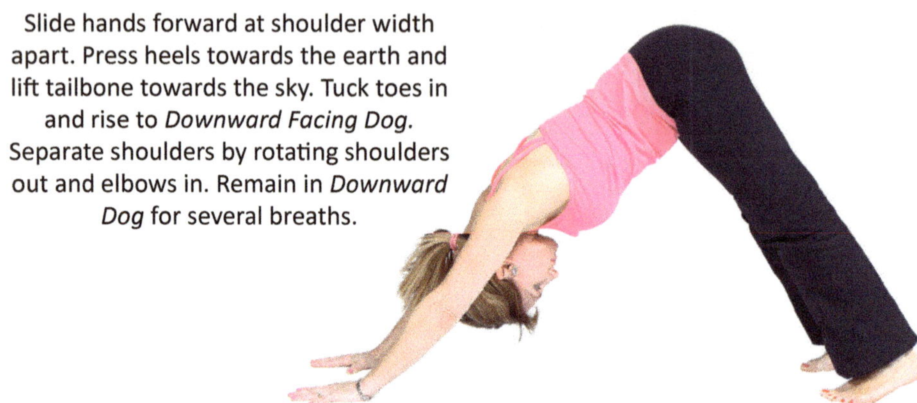

PLANK

Increases core strength, chest and arms.

From *Downward Dog*, breathe into *Plank pose* On hands and toes, lift belly button in, contract pelvic floor muscle and hold.

If you have spinal injuries, back pain, or if you need to build strength, begin *Plank* on your knees until strength improves.

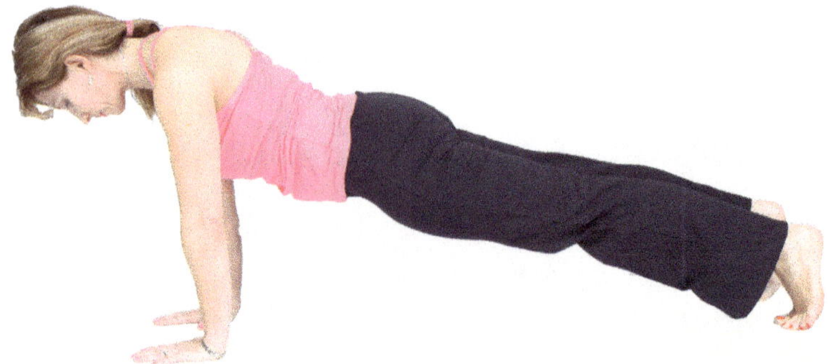

From toes or knees; remain in Plank for up to thirty seconds before moving into *Crocodile pose*.

CROCODILE POSE

From *Plank pose*, breathe out to *Crocodile pose*. Lower your body in a one way push up, hold above mat for five to ten seconds before resting on the floor. An option is to add ten push-ups to increase strength. *Crocodile pose* can be done from your toes (as in a full push up) or from your knees. From *Crocodile pose*, breathe in to *Up-Dog*.

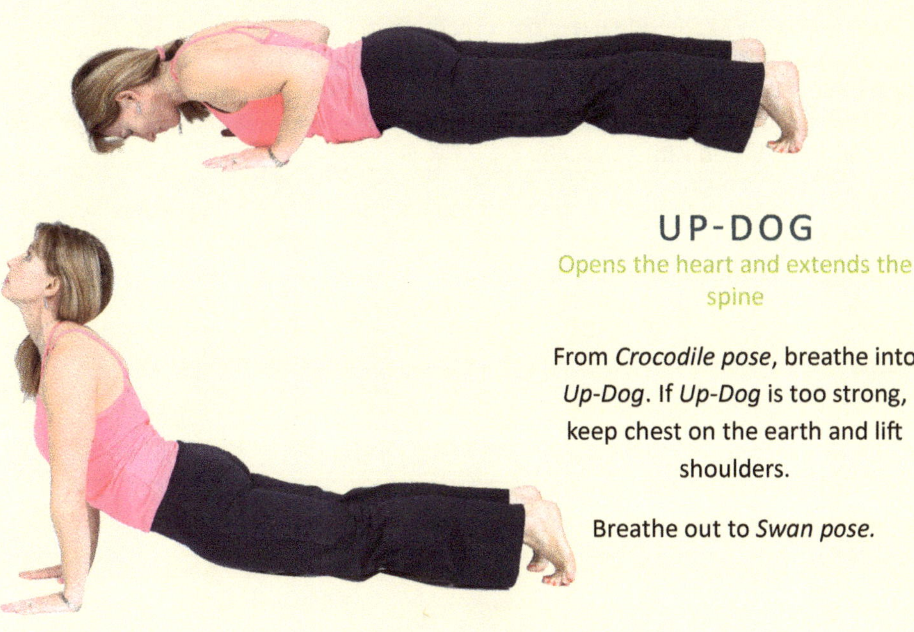

UP-DOG

From *Crocodile pose*, breathe into *Up-Dog*. If *Up-Dog* is too strong, keep chest on the earth and lift shoulders.

Breathe out to *Swan pose*.

SWAN POSE

Press bottom to heels and lengthen spine. Tuck in chin and tail bone. Lengthen arms.

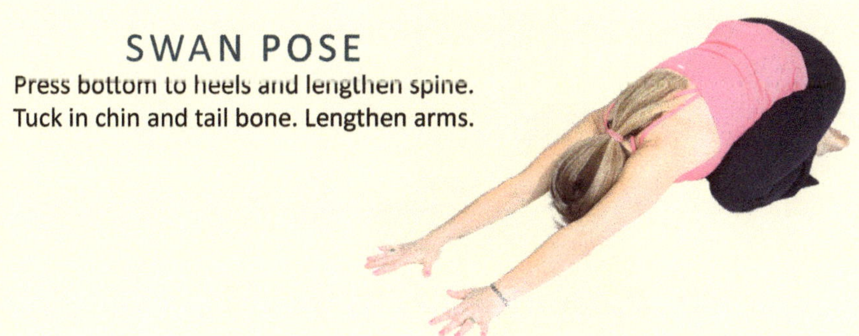

Repeat this rythmic pattern for several rounds.

Finish in *Child's pose*.

Head of a Cow

Releases shoulders and hips

I used to wonder how this could possibly be a head of a cow? Then a friend showed me - the knees represent the cow's lips, and the arms their ears. Ahuh! Head of a Cow stretches hips, shoulders and more. Softer options are to sit cross-legged, with arms folded behind back.

Don't worry if you can't do every posture, that's life. We start where we are, and with acceptance and grace, we move towards where we want to be. Whilst you're in this pose (or any pose) breathe deeply and let go of expectations. Tune into the tightness and say to yourself 'I accept myself, just as I am.' The tightness will begin to dissolve. All tightness began with a thought.

The most common thought is 'I'm not good enough.' By reminding yourself that you are good enough and acceptable, just as you are, your body lets go, your mind lets go, and flexibility and peace move in.

Begin in cross-legged for option one, or cross one leg over the top and wrap feet around for option two.

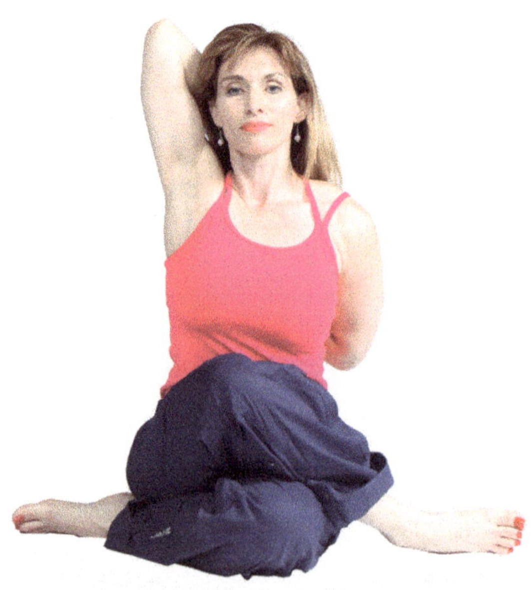

Love, honour and accept yourself, just as you are, right now.

HEAD OF A COW
option one

Fold arms behind back for option one.

Press heart forward and roll shoulders back. When you change sides, remember to place the other arm on top.

HEAD OF A COW
option two

Bring one arm to the top and the other arm wrapped around back, Press lower hand reaching up as the other hand reaches down. Monkey grip when they meet. Press shoulders back and heart to sky.

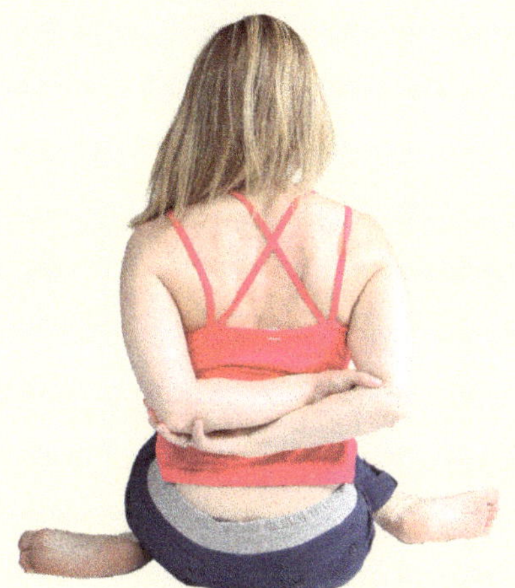

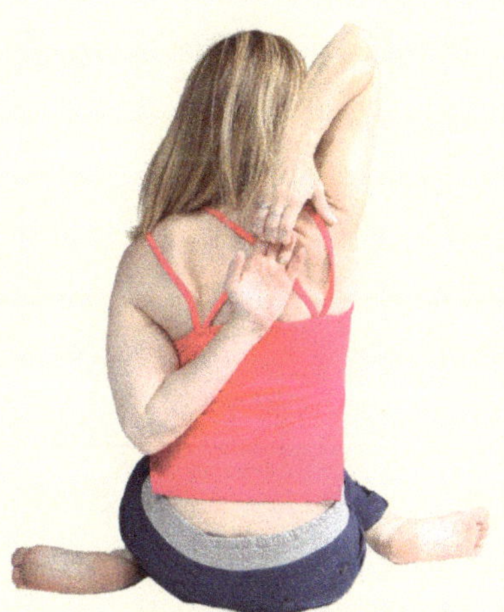

Lengthen the spine and breathe. Let go of tension.

Hold for one minute, release gently, and change sides

'Thoughts make up your world.
Good thoughts lead to good days.
Good days lead to good weeks.
Good weeks lead to good months
Good months lead to good years.'

Bert Weir

fun

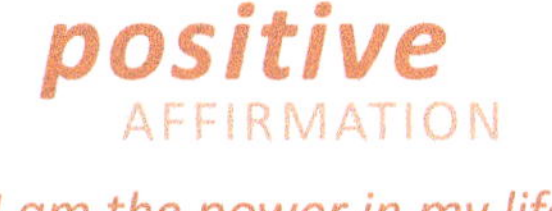

positive
AFFIRMATION
I am the power in my life

humour

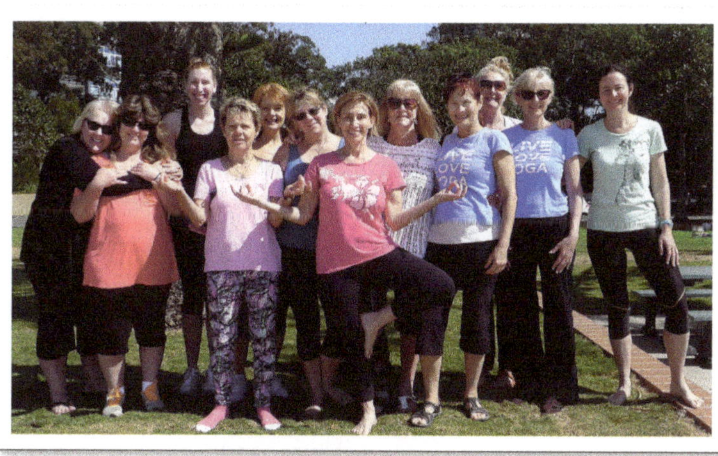

positive
AFFIRMATION

I find my tribe and we find each other

creativity

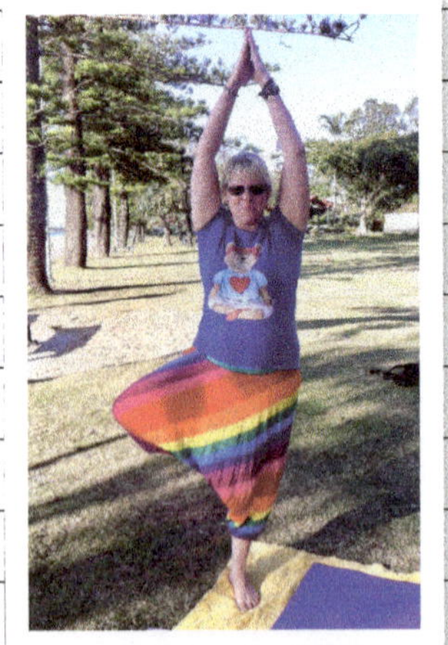

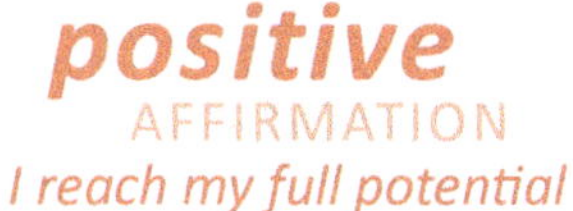

positive
AFFIRMATION
I reach my full potential

integrity

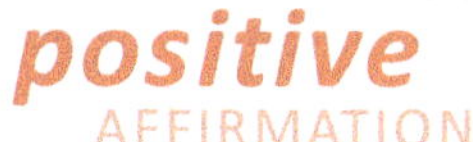

positive
AFFIRMATION

I respect myself, and I choose my own values

A Rhythmic Pattern
From Mountain pose to Half Moon

Begin in *Mountain pose.*

Breathe in and reach back, breathe out to *Forward Fold.*

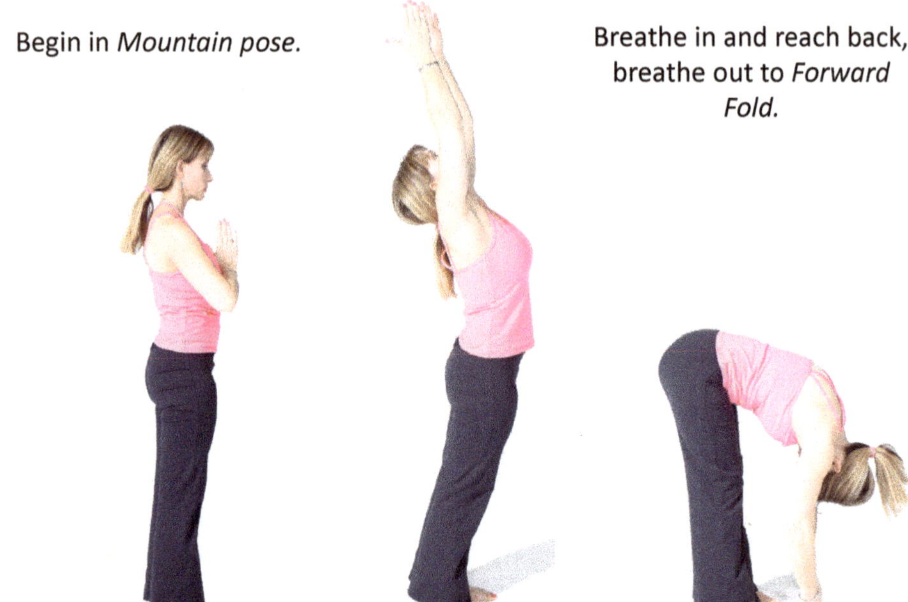

Breathe in and place hands onto the earth, breathe out to step back to *Downward Dog*.

Breathe in to lift the right leg for *Three Legged Dog*, and scoop right foot between hands for a *Lunge*.

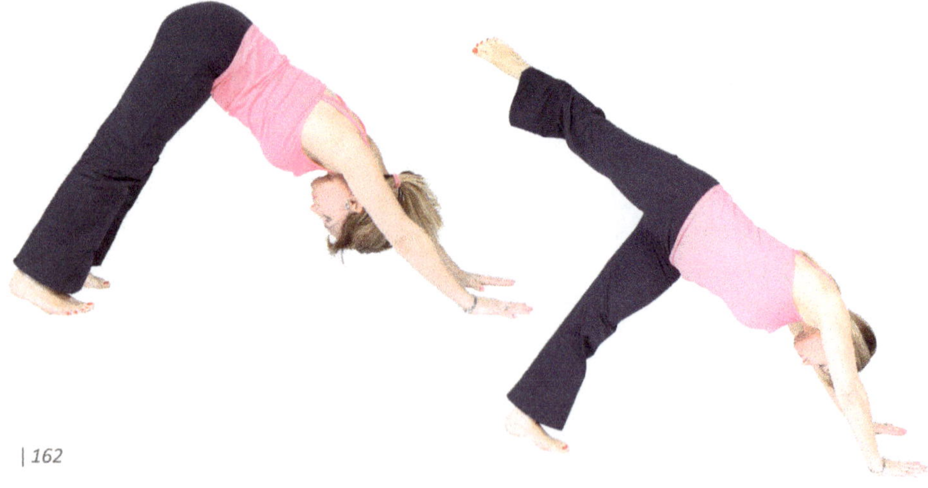

From *Lunge,* softly rise, keep the weight on the front leg as you slowly lift into *Aeroplane pose*. Keep the foot on the earth for option one, lift the leg for option two. Stretch the arms out. Breathe.

From *Aeroplane pose*, tilt left hand towards the earth and right hand towards the sky for *Half Moon Pose*.

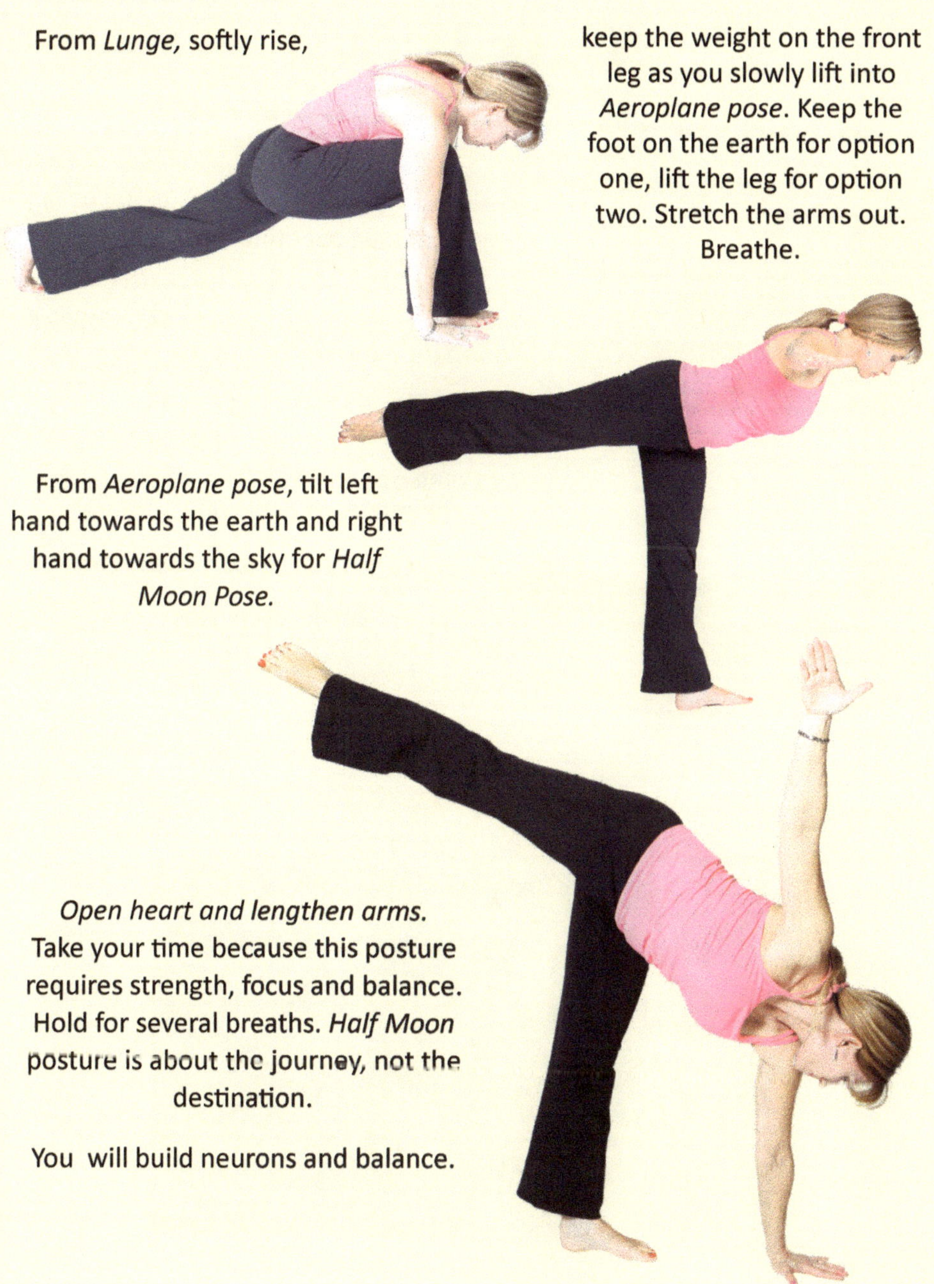

Open heart and lengthen arms. Take your time because this posture requires strength, focus and balance. Hold for several breaths. *Half Moon* posture is about the journey, not the destination.

You will build neurons and balance.

From *Half Moon*, bring back foot beside front foot, bend both knees, breathe in and softly rise, breathe out bring hands to heart. Pause. Change sides.

WILD THING

You make my heart sing

OPTION ONE

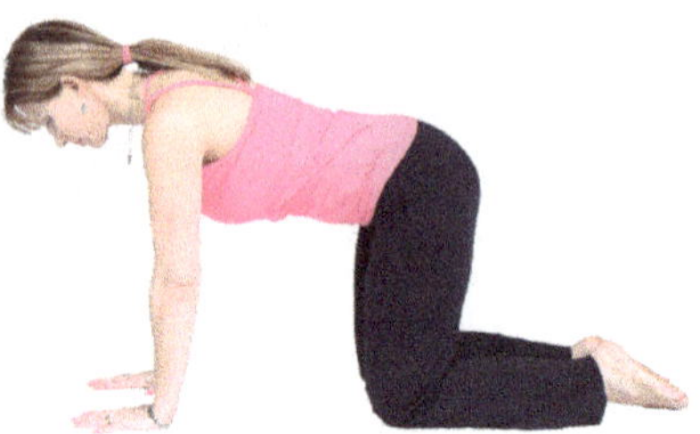

From hands and knees, lift right leg to sky. Reach right leg over until your foot touches the earth.

Keep left knee on the earth as you slowly lift your right hand to sky and reach arm back.

Hold for several breaths.

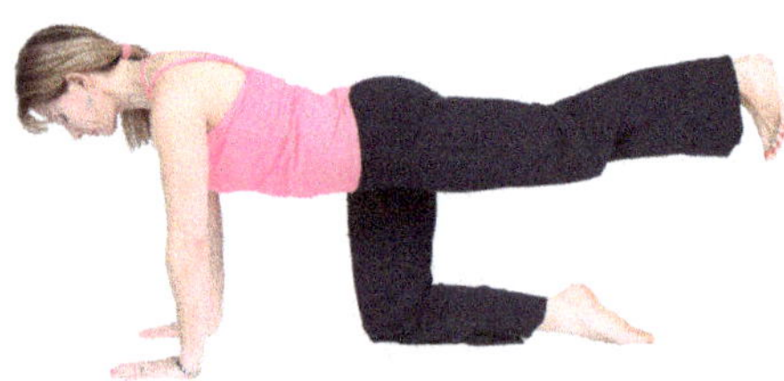

Come out of *Wild Thing* by reversing the moves of how you got there.

Rest in *Child's pose* for a few breaths.

Do the other side.

Become a Wild Thing!

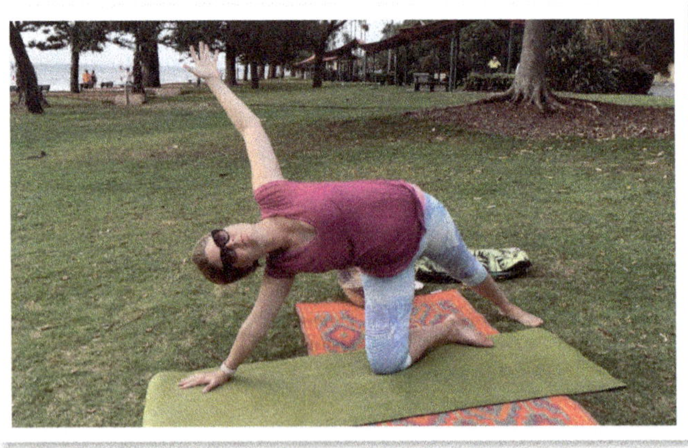

If *Wild Thing* is too much for you, just sing the song, and you will experience the benefits anyway.

Enjoy your wild and happy self!

WILD THING

I think I love you

OPTION TWO

Begin in *Downward Dog*. Step feet forward
one step, so that heels are on the earth
(this will help you stay balanced).

Lift right leg to sky for *Three-Legged Dog*.
Lengthen leg away from your body until it is over
the other side, and plant foot onto earth.

Adjust feet so they are balanced.
Press hips up to the sky.

Lift right arm up towards the sky. Come out of
pose by reversing the moves of how you got
there.

Rest in *Child's pose* for a few breaths.

Do the other side.

Become a Wild Thing!

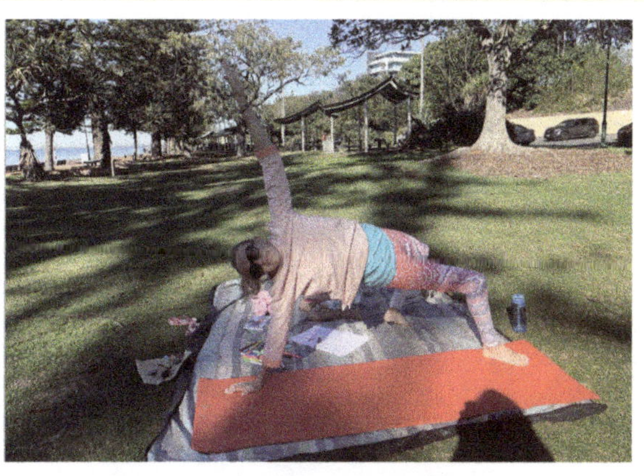

Tune into You.

Always do postures with the utmost respect for your body.

Wild and Free. That is Me.

gratitude

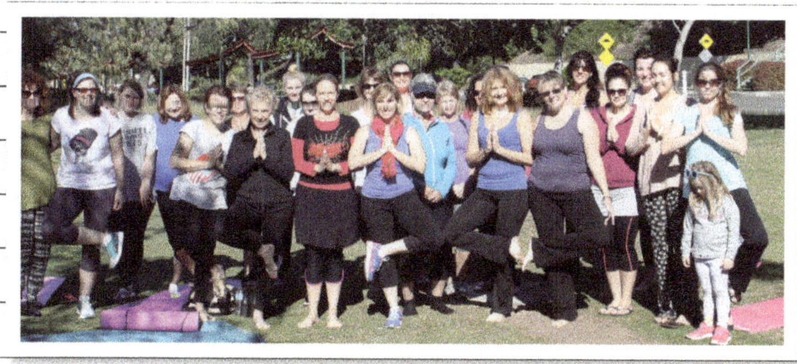

positive
AFFIRMATION

I love all of me, just as I am

generous

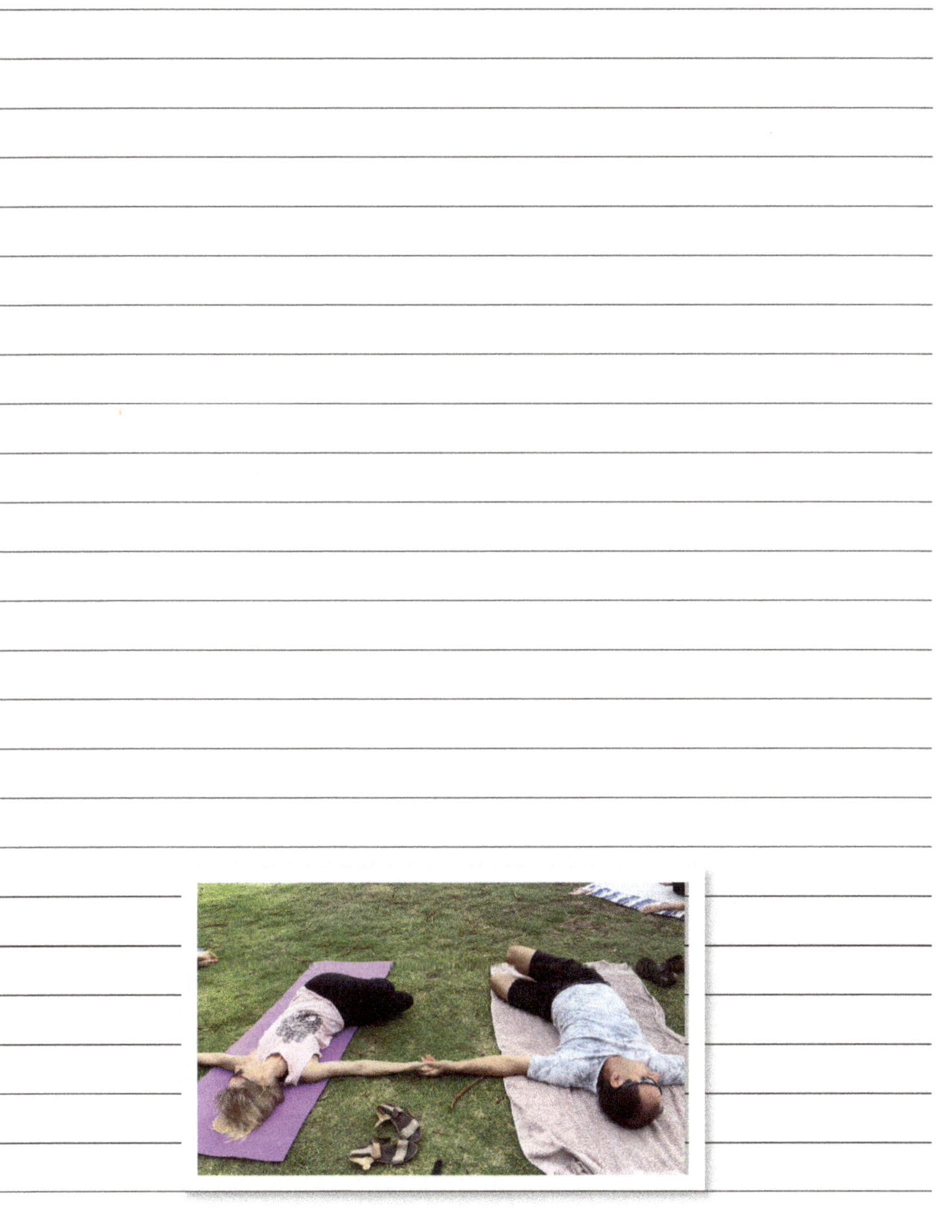

positive
AFFIRMATION

Flexible, creative, purposeful, wonderful, me

grace

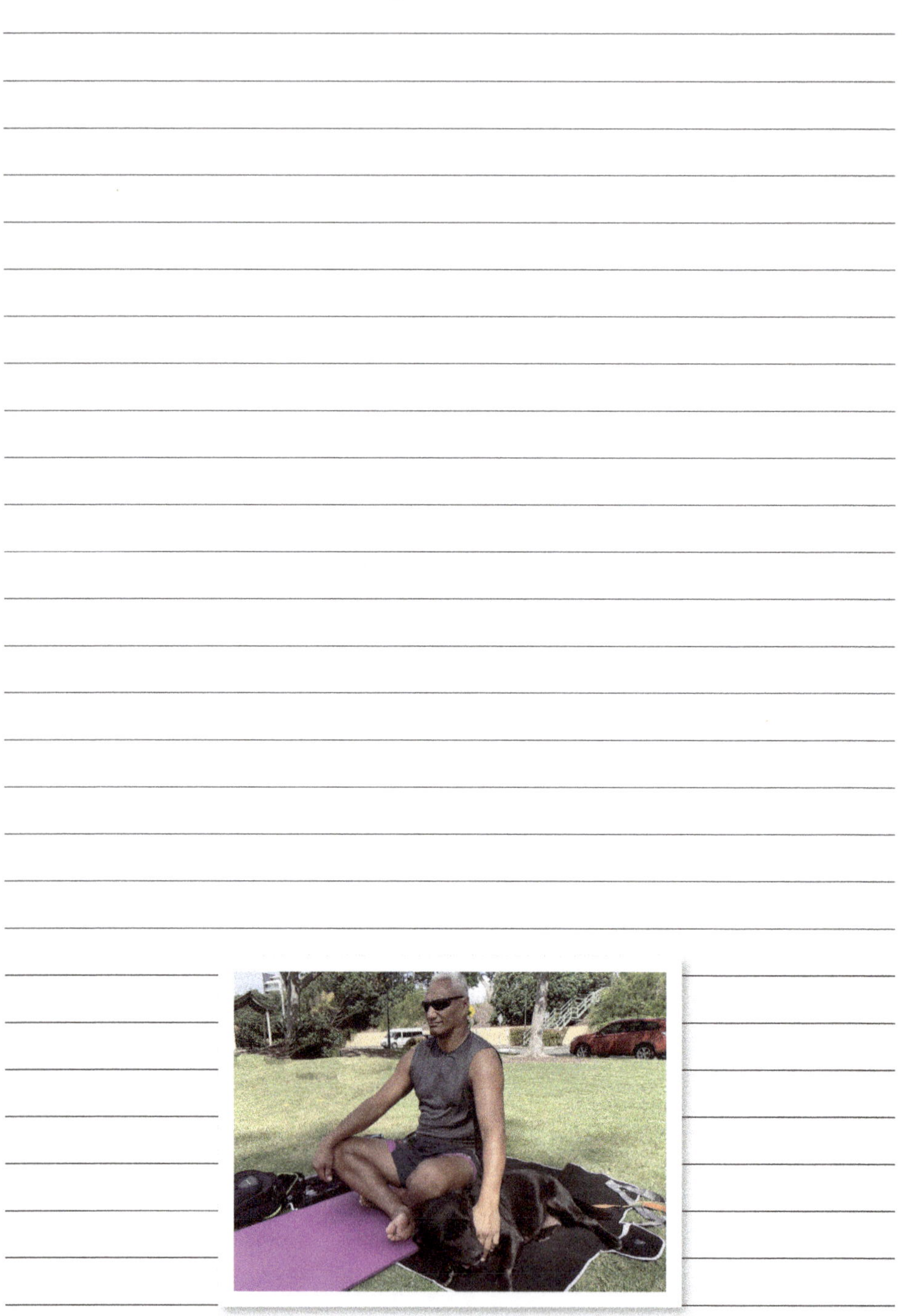

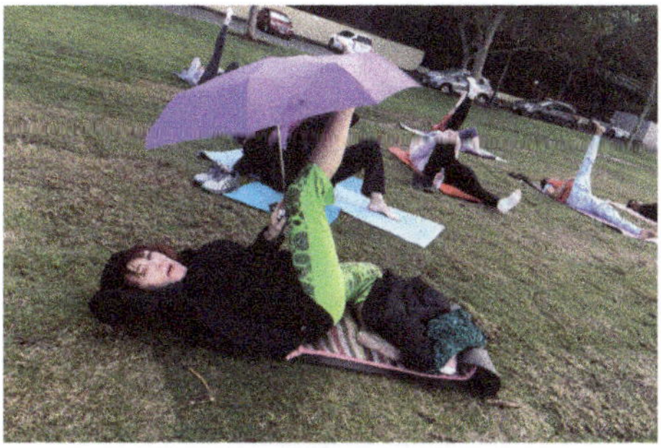

positive
AFFIRMATION

I am flexible in mind, body, spirit

empathy

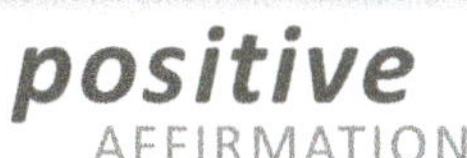

positive
AFFIRMATION

I look for the good in myself and others

Gate Pose, Side Plank & Star Pose

GATE POSE

Kneel and extend right leg. Keep hips pressed forward and aligned. Lengthen body and breathe in, raise left arm to sky, and as you breathe out reach across, and slide along the outstretched leg for *Gate pose*.

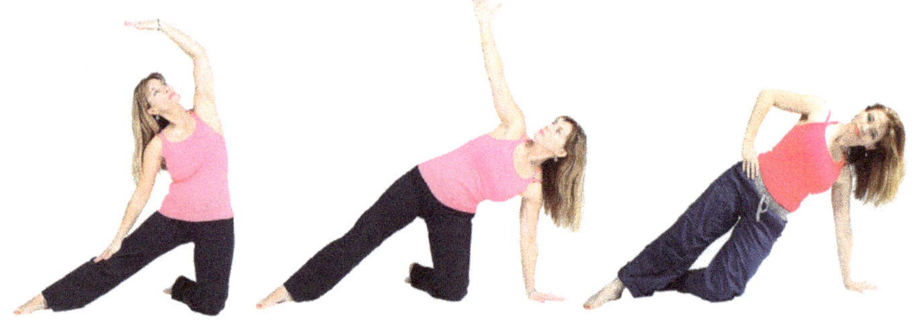

SIDE PLANK

From *Gate pose*, move the top arm to place on the earth beneath shoulder. Stay here for option one. Extend lower leg for option two, or take both feet onto the earth into *Side Plank* for option three. Lift the waist. Lift the arm. Lift pelvic floor. Breathe.

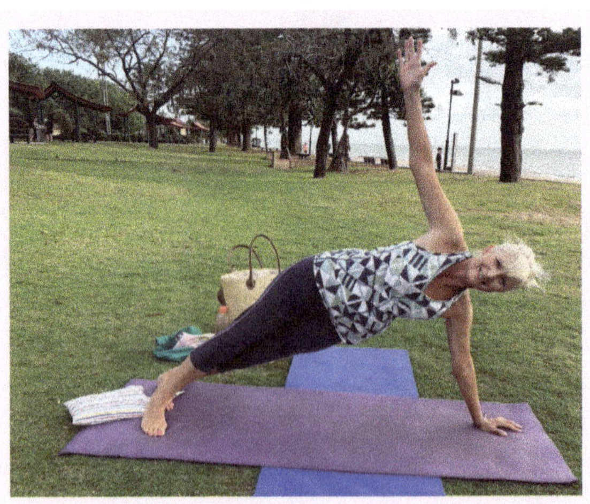

SIDE STAR

From *Side Plank*, lift the top leg and
become a beautiful *Star*.

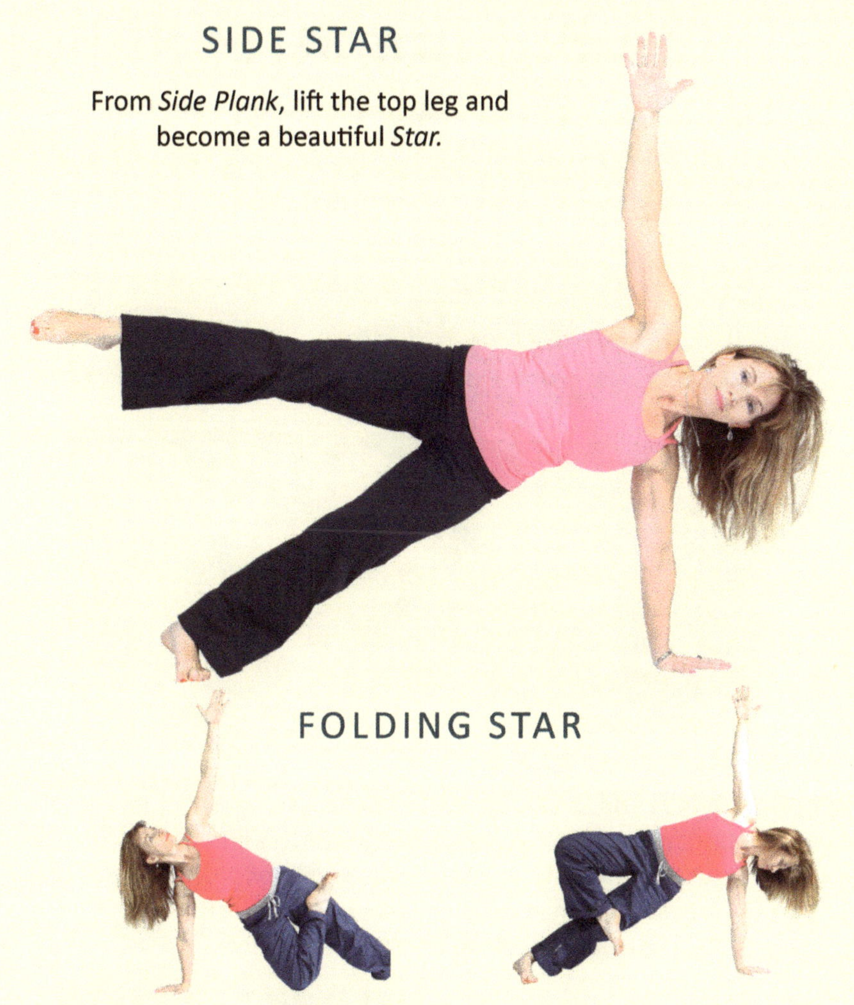

FOLDING STAR

Side Star leads naturally into *Folding Star*. From *Side Star*, you can fold the top
leg down, or the lower leg up. Keep hips high, take lower knee to earth for
a softer option. Hold each posture for up to one minute. Rest in *Child's pose*
before changing sides. *Gate, Side Plank, Star* and *Side Star* strengthen the core,
hips, shoulders and legs.

The possibilities for variations are endless. We could stay here all day like a
Marconi set, moving our bodies into different shapes. The most important
thing to remember in yoga (and in life) is to go with your body.
Teach your body to trust you. Take yourself to the edge and ease
yourself into postures with love and acceptance, just as you would in life.

The Big Toe Stretch

You will love the benefits of this pose. *Yes it hurt*s, but, when you find you can bounce higher, run faster and *relieve athritis in your toes*, you're going to love it.

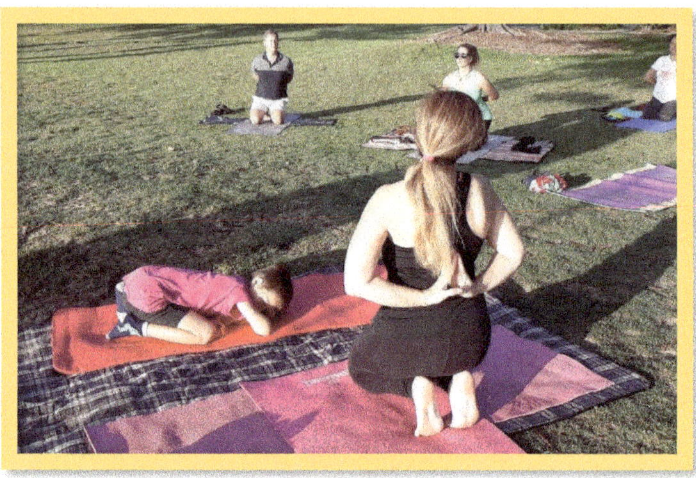

Begin on your hands and knees. Tuck all of the toes under. Adjust knees wider to help. Option one, keep your hands on the earth and press bottom back towards toes. Option two, sit on heels and bring hands in *Reverse Namaste*. Breathe. Smile. Smiling increases endorphins and endorphins are a natural pain reliever.

A local pre-natal group includes the Big Toe Stretch in their yoga class to help women breathe through intense experiences.

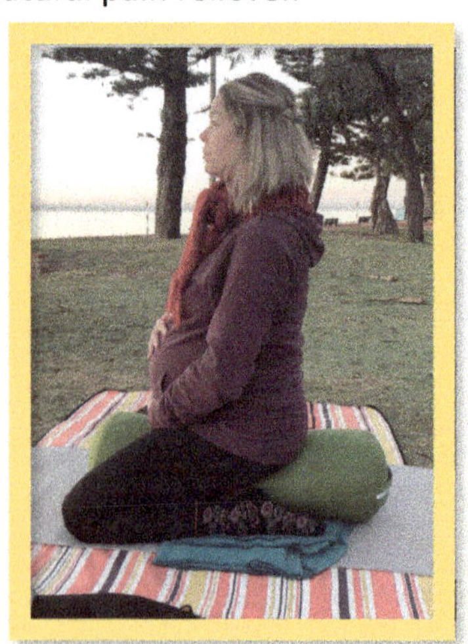

Find Your Self

I am where I am, and it's enough

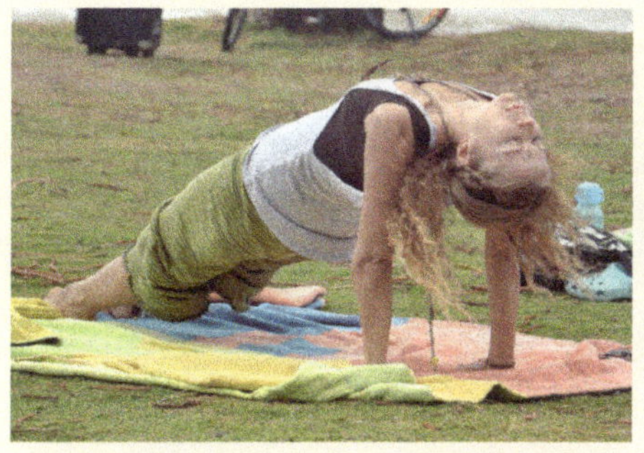

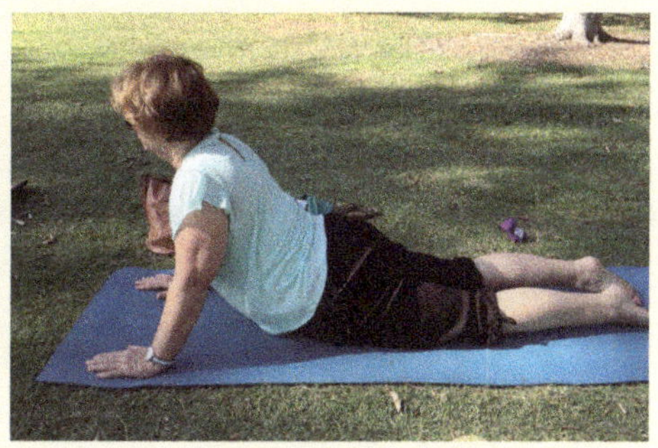

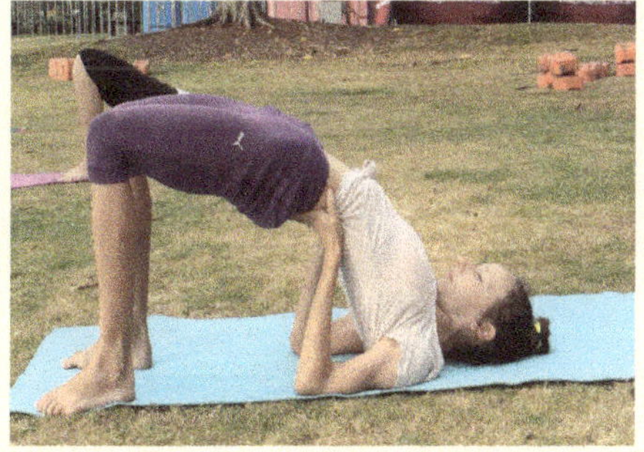

I already have all of the skills and talent that I need to move towards my greatest good and highest joy

I am already perfect, whole and complete. All I need to do is to tune into my breath and accept who I am

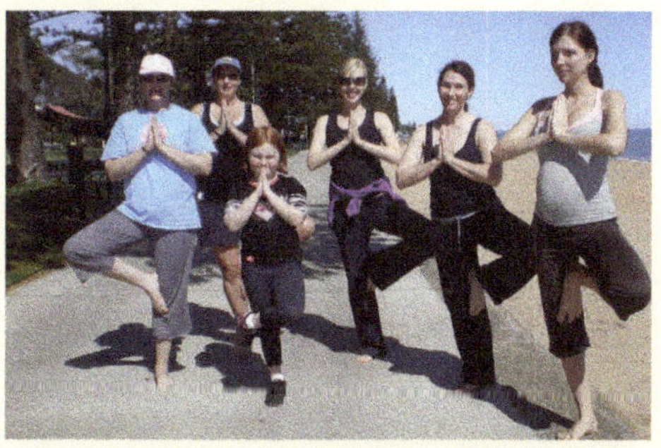

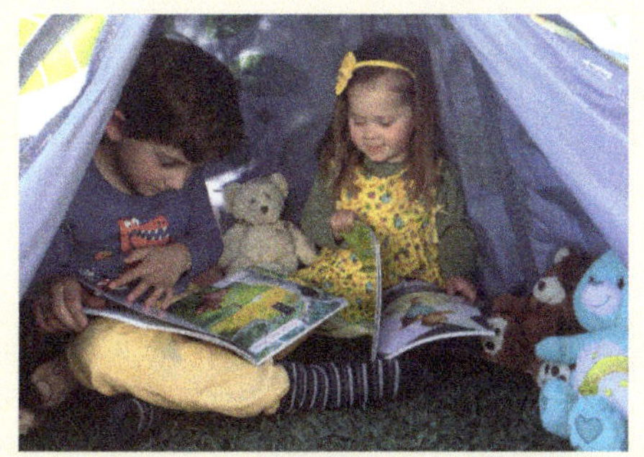

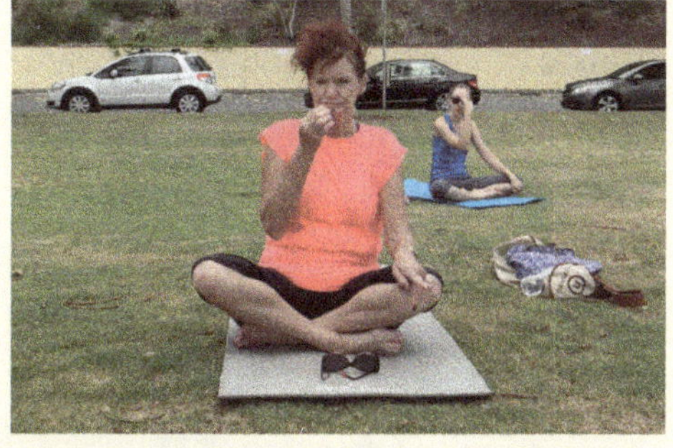

Yoga Dogs

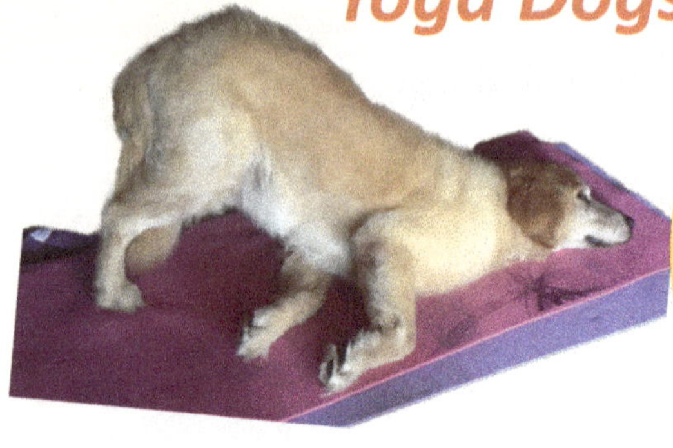

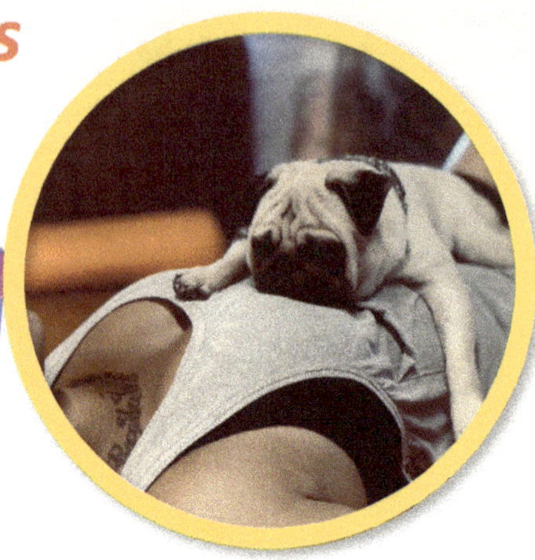

Family friendly yoga

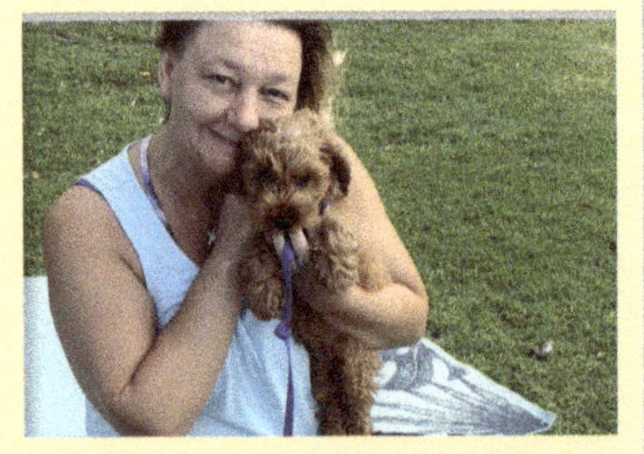

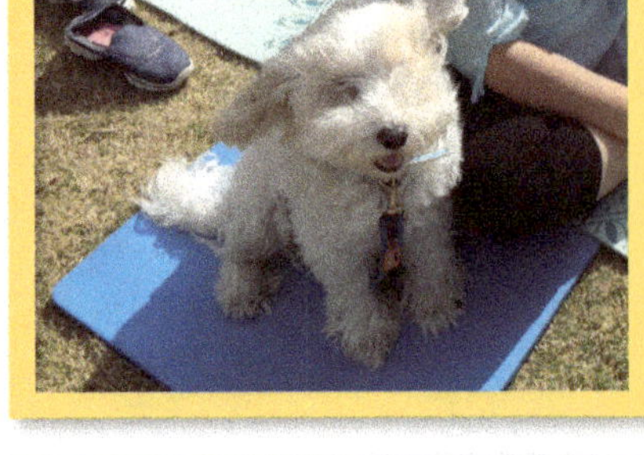

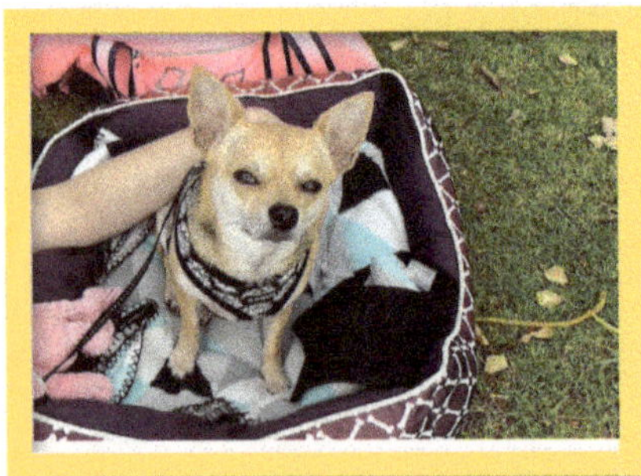

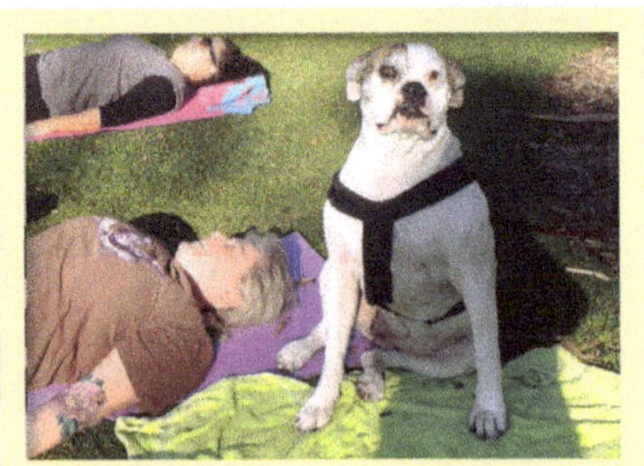

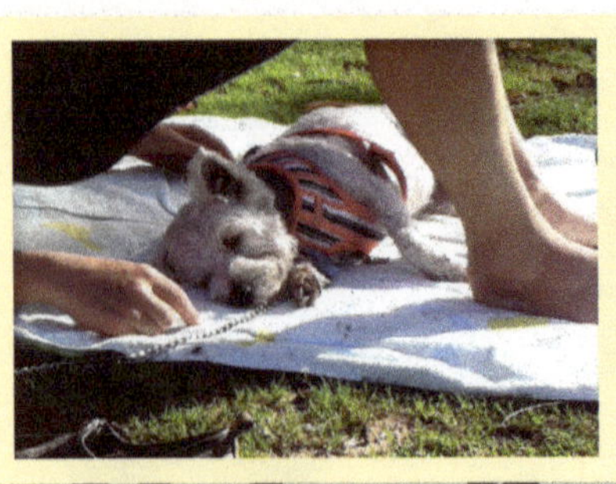

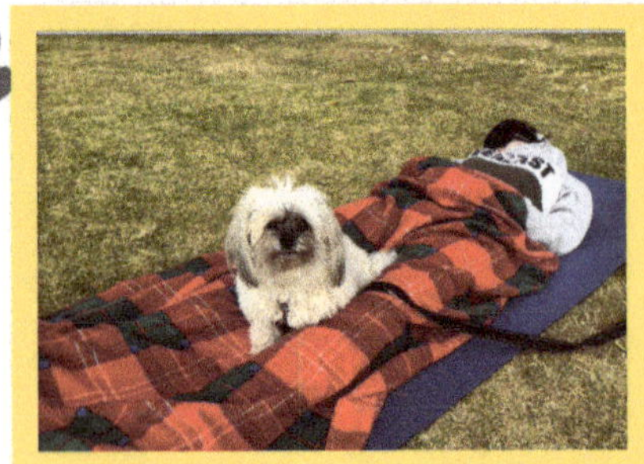

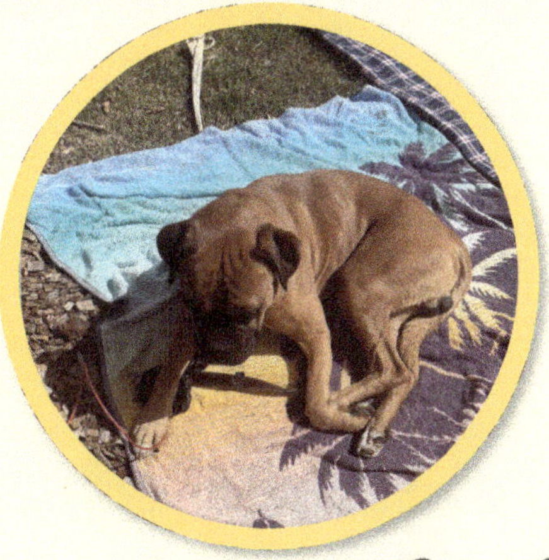

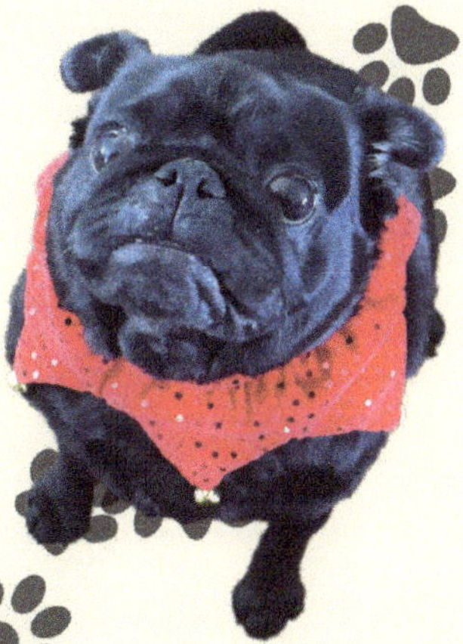

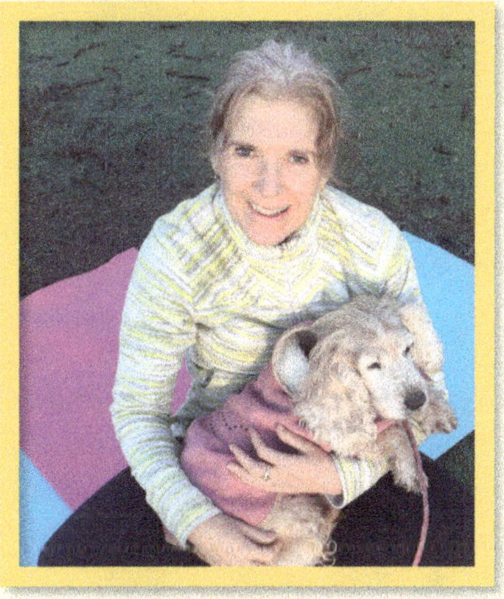

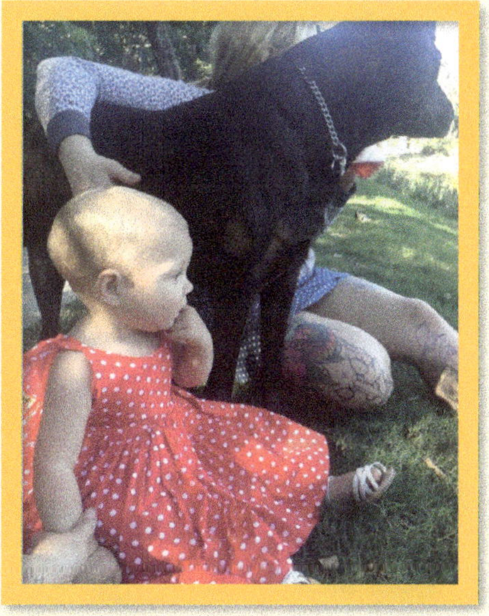

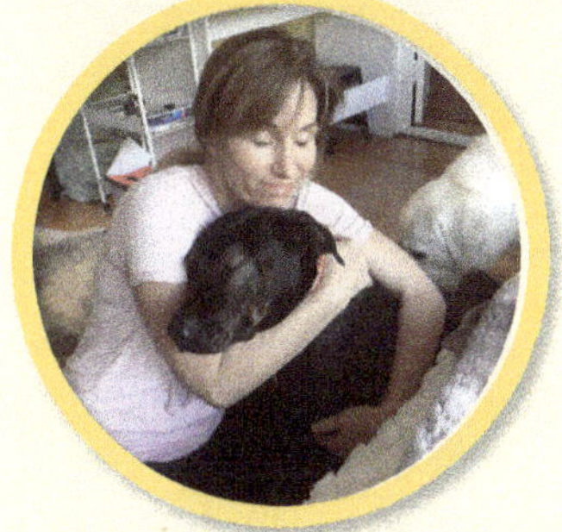
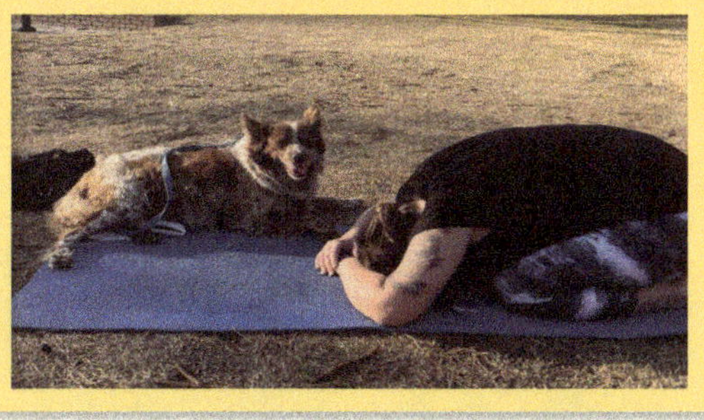

friendly

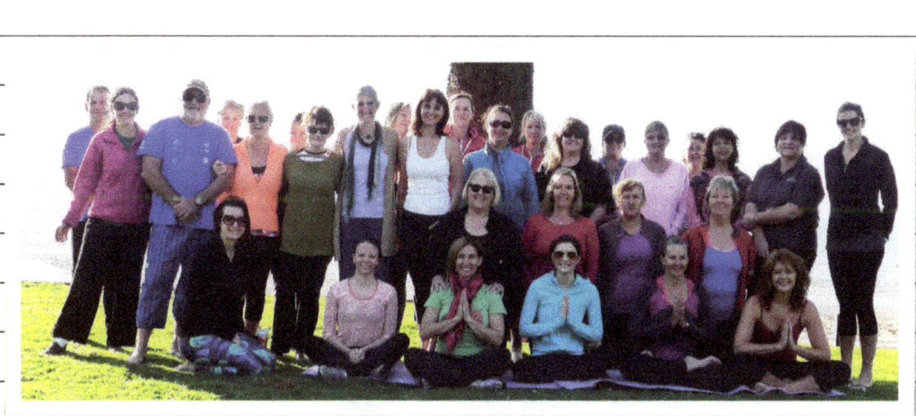

positive
AFFIRMATION

I am doing the very best that I can

imagine

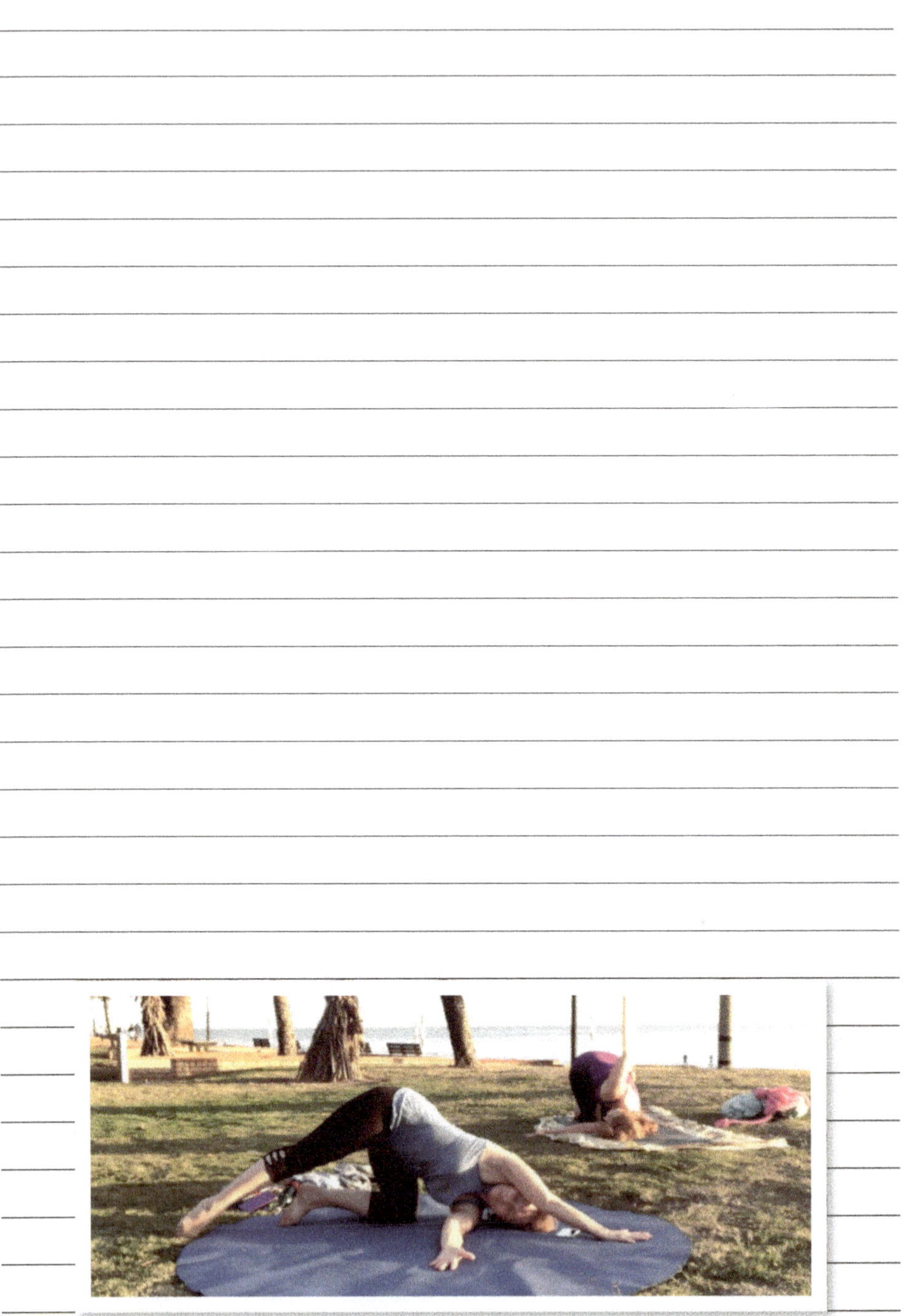

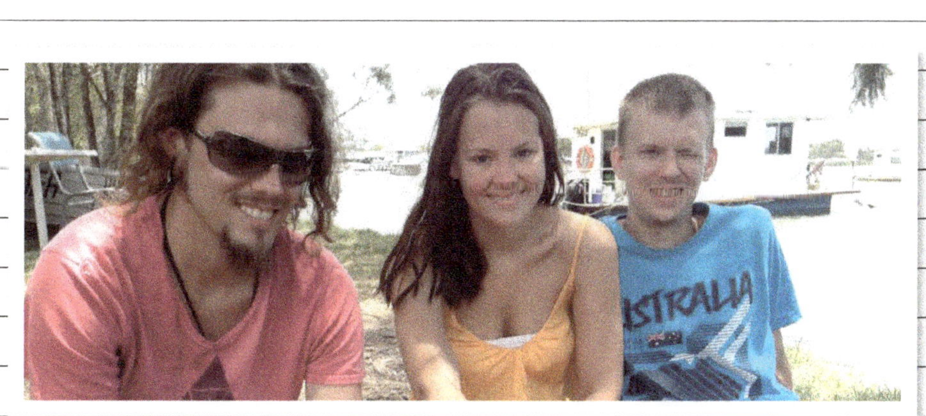

positive
AFFIRMATION

I find peace where ever I go

dream

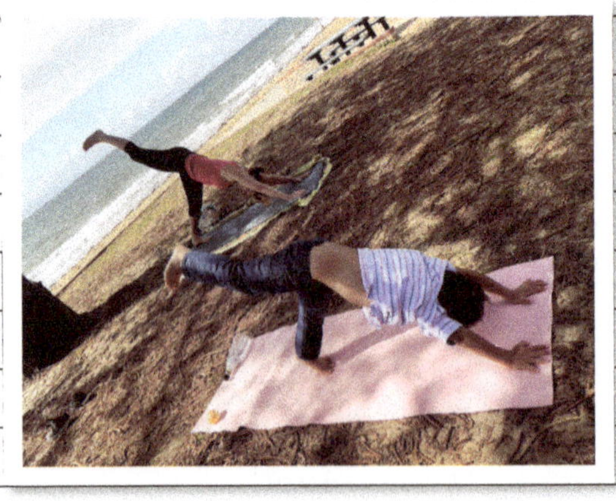

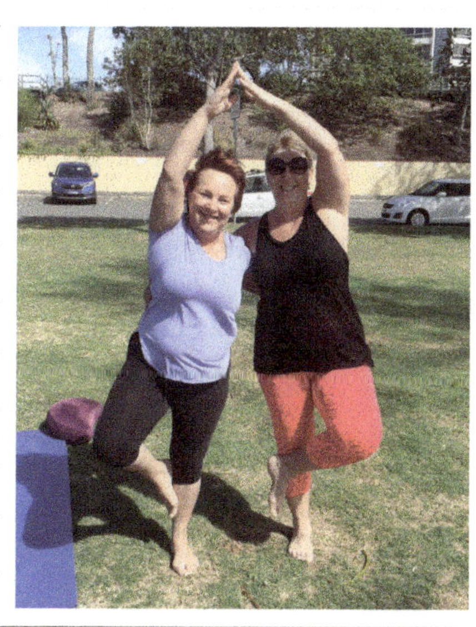

positive
AFFIRMATION

I am thankful for all of the good in my life

believe

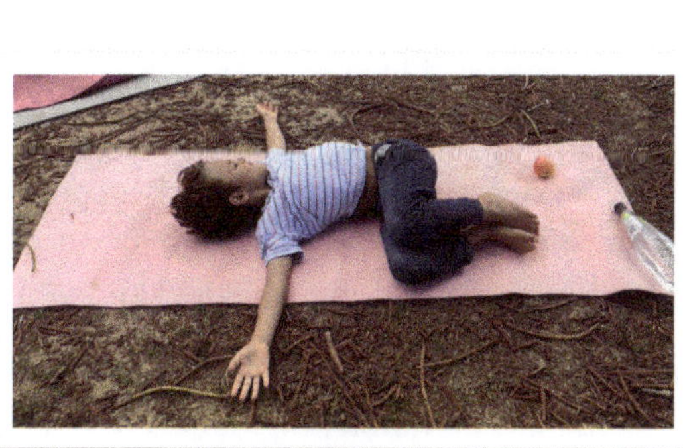

positive
AFFIRMATION

I love myself, I love my life, I make positive choices

PELVIC ROCK
Strengthens pelvic floor

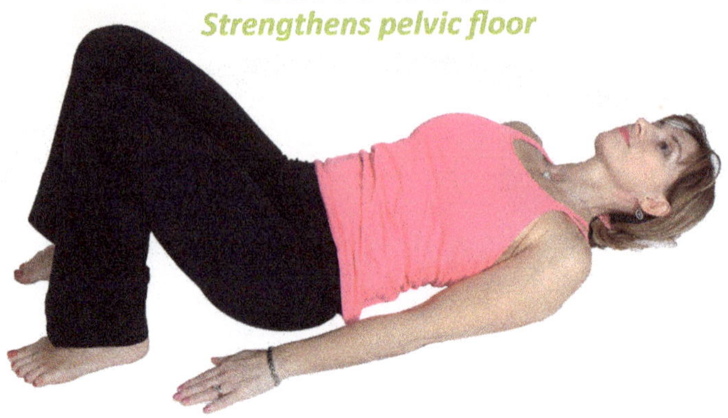

The *pelvic floor* is the muscle that slings between the pubic bone and the tail bone. A strong pelvic floor will gift you with the confidence to run, skip, hop and bounce. It will enhance your sexuality and improve your posture. You can do pelive floor contractions anytime, anywhere.

Lay on the mat with knees bent. Lengthen spine and rest arms by side.
Keep feet, hips and shoulders in the same line.
Breathe into tummy and lengthen the exhale.
Breathe in, open the ribs and as you exhale, press lower back towards the earth, tilt tailbone up and contract (or squeeze) the pelvic floor muscle.
Breathe in; release, breathe out; squeeze and contract.
Repeat ten times. If you're not sure where the pelvic floor muscle is, imagine you are trying to stop a wee—the muscle you use to pull up is your pelvic floor. For guys, lift your testes. Once you know where your pelvic floor muscle is you can do this exercise anywhere (and no-one will know).

BRIDGE POSE
Strength and Boost

From *Pelvic Rock* we move into *Bridge Pose.*
Bridge pose stimulates the thyroid to produce thyroxin,
which boosts metabolism and immunity.
Bridge pose strengthens lower back, gluteus and hamstrings.
You can do up to three *Bridge pose*s, making each one stronger than the last, or stay in option one for each round.
Begin in neutral position.
Option one; Keep feet, hip and shoulders in alignment. Inhale, and as you exhale, press lower back towards the earth, lift pelvic floor, peel spine off the earth and press hips to sky. Hold for up to 30 seconds.

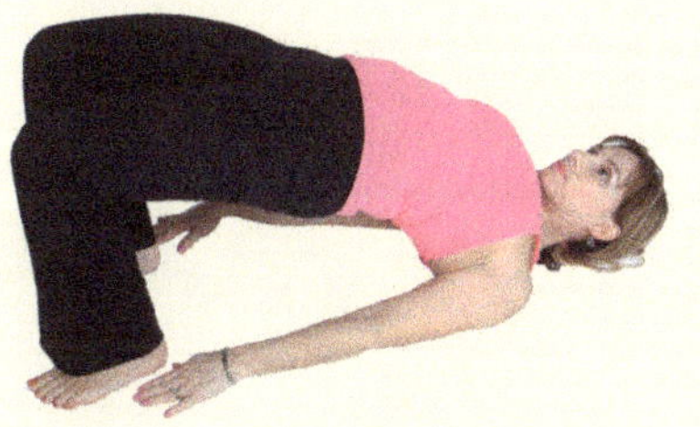 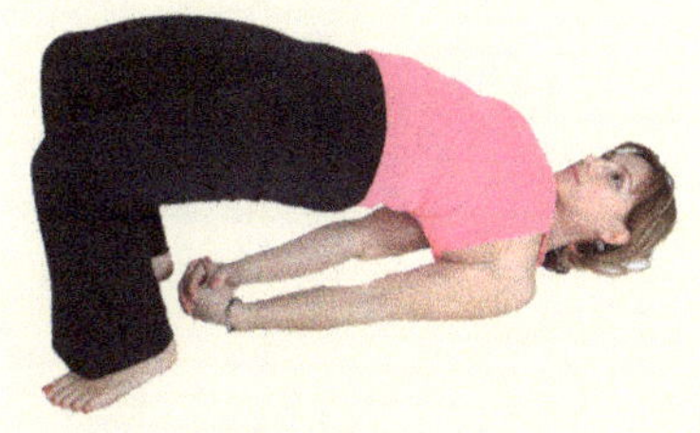

Bring knees to chest and press. Repeat *Bridge pose.* For option two; roll onto shoulders, clasp hands underneath and press. For option three; place hands to hips and press up to sky. Opiton four is *Wheel pose.* If you have any back issues that may be impacted by *Wheel pose*, stay with option one or two.

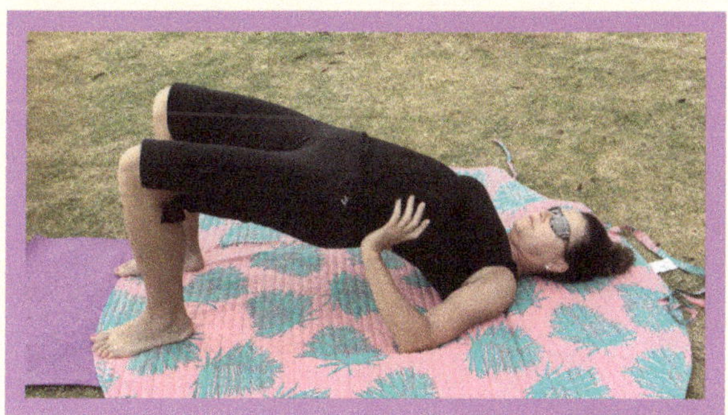

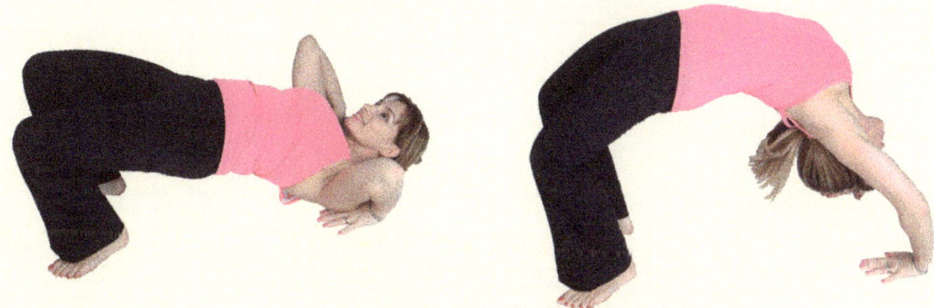

WHEEL POSE
An advanced option

From *Bridge pose*, reach hands beneath shoulders and press up. Keep feet firm, knees in alignment with hips and squeeze gluteus. Press hips to sky. Hold until your body says 'enough'. That might only be a few seconds or a minute. When you are ready, lay your head down first and gently return your spine to the earth. Finish with a *Beach Ball* and move into a *Free Choice Back roll.*

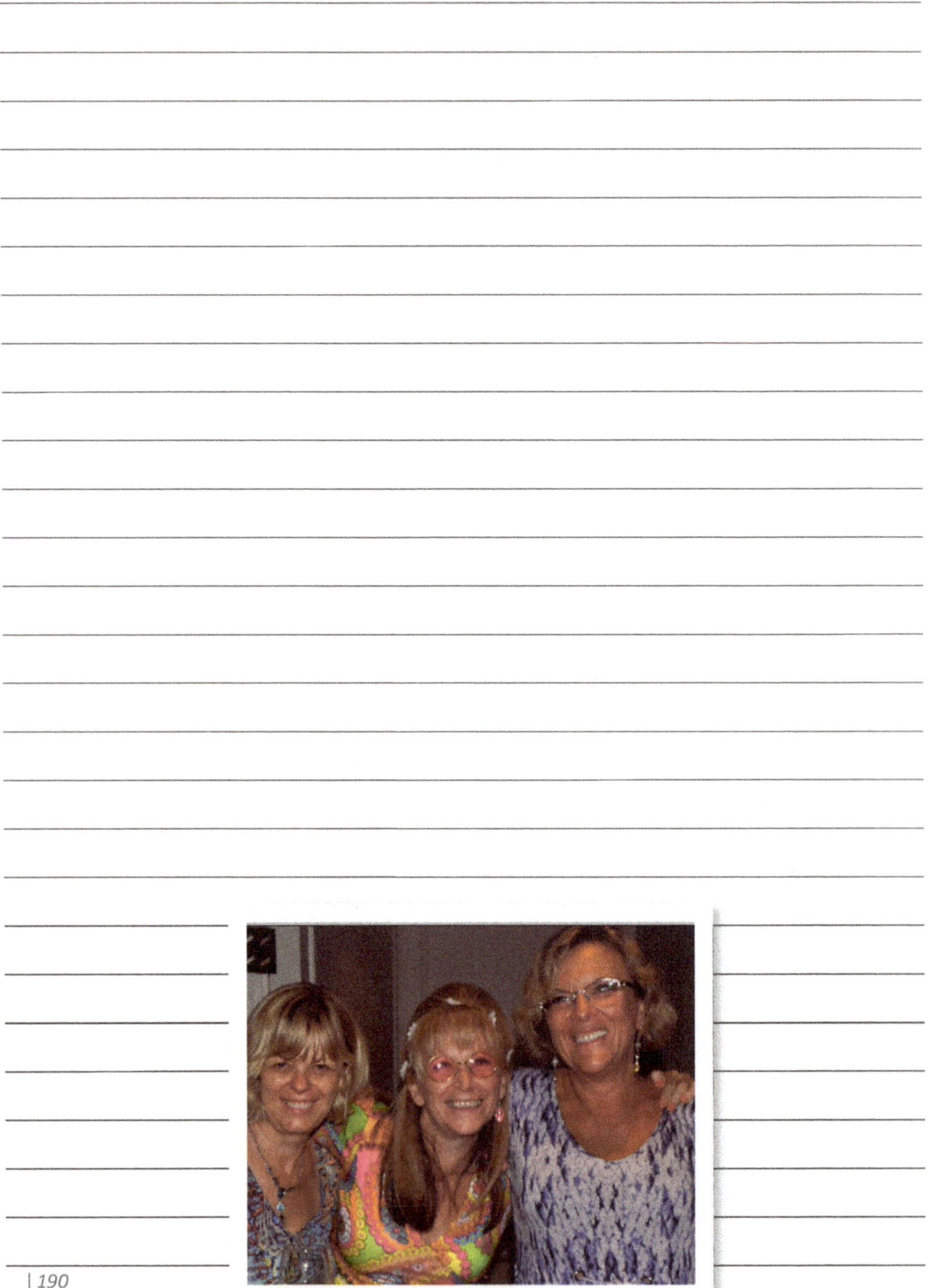

positive
AFFIRMATION

It is what it is, I am where I am

trust

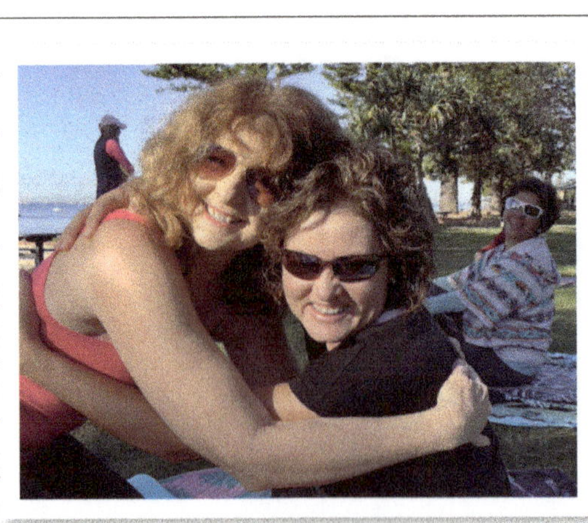

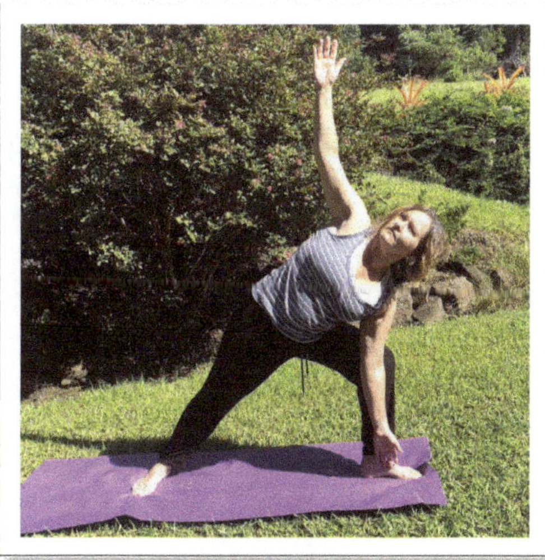

positive
AFFIRMATION
And where I am is good, because, it's where I am

acceptance

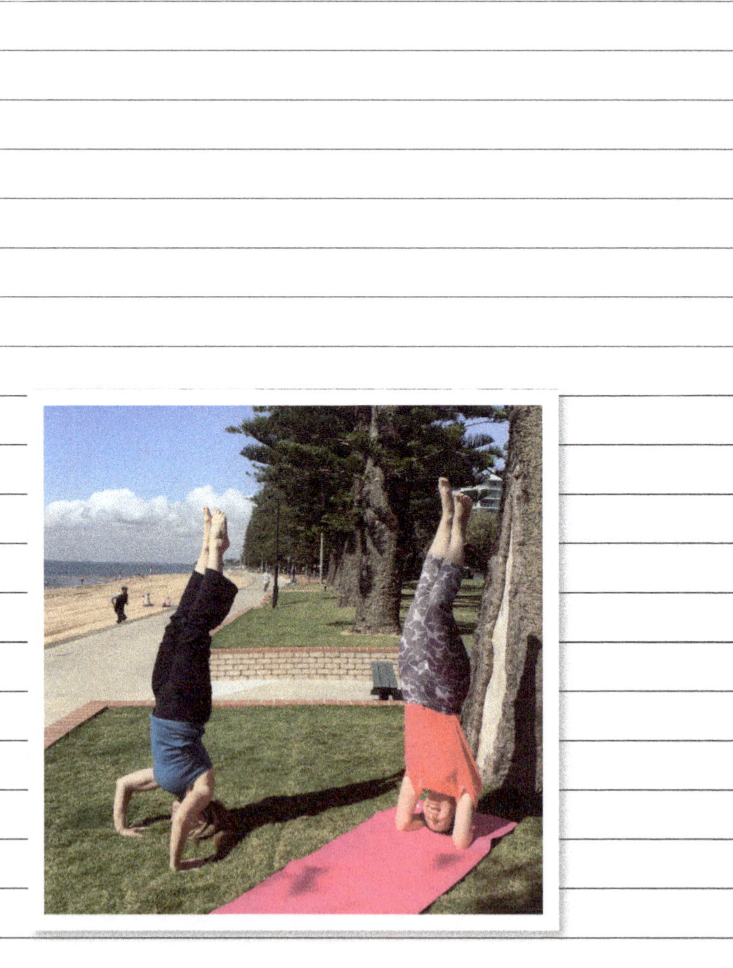

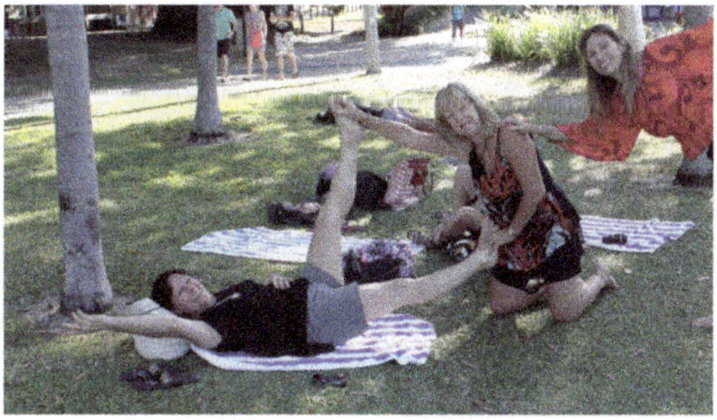

positive
AFFIRMATION

Acceptance helps me move forward

faith

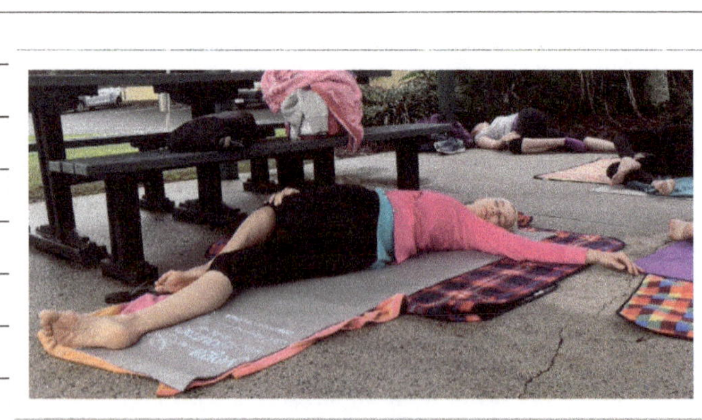

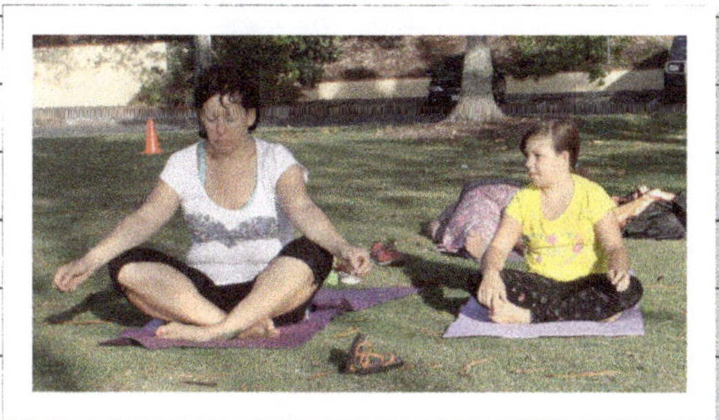

positive
AFFIRMATION
I am awesome

FREE CHOICE BACK ROLLS
Rock and Roll in any way that serves your back.

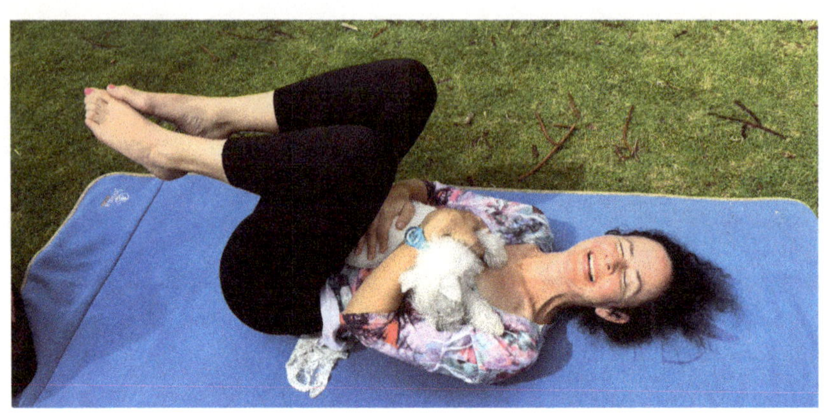

SPINAL TWIST

Lay on the earth. Breathe in and stretch the whole body. As you exhale, bring right knee to chest, press. Hold for a few breaths. Place left hand to knee and take this leg over to the right side. Relax. Adjust shoulders. Breathe into your back. Breathe deeply.

Two minutes of *Spinal Twist* will do wonders for your spine.

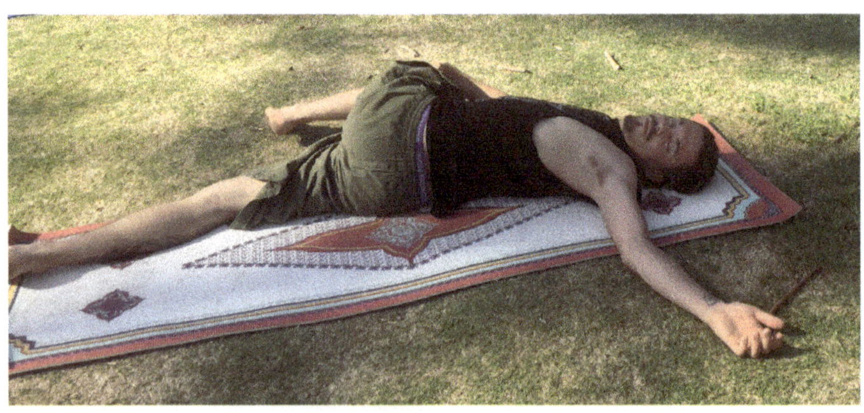

FREE CHOICE
From *Spinal Twist* move into *Free Choice*.
Free Choice is whatever you need.
From *Free Choice* we move into *Meditation*.

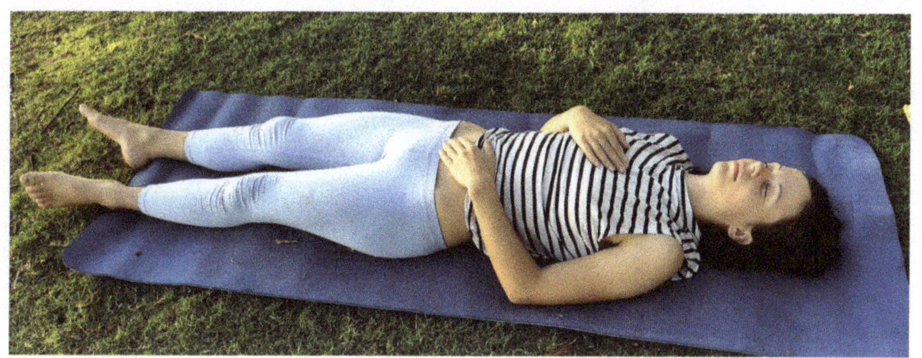

Meditation

Some of the benefits of meditation are lower blood pressure, lower stress, higher immunity and a better memory.

Play ambient music. Lie in *Peaceful pose*, or sit in comfortable cross-legged position. Take several deep breaths and release all tension. Focus on your breath and become aware of how your breath moves in and out of your body.

As thoughts enter your mind, let them go and return to your breath. Take deep breaths, and with each exhale, release and relax every muscle.

As you feel your breath becoming quiet and slow, focus on your toes and consciously relax each one. Relax each muscle from the toes to the feet, to the ankles, breathing deeply; release your calves, shins, thighs and hamstrings.

Let your body go, bring your awareness back to your breath. Focus on your breath as you breathe in and out.

Relax hips, abdomen and chest. Let yourself soften. Let go of your shoulders, arms and hands. Soften upper back, middle back, lower back and gluteus. *Breathe...*

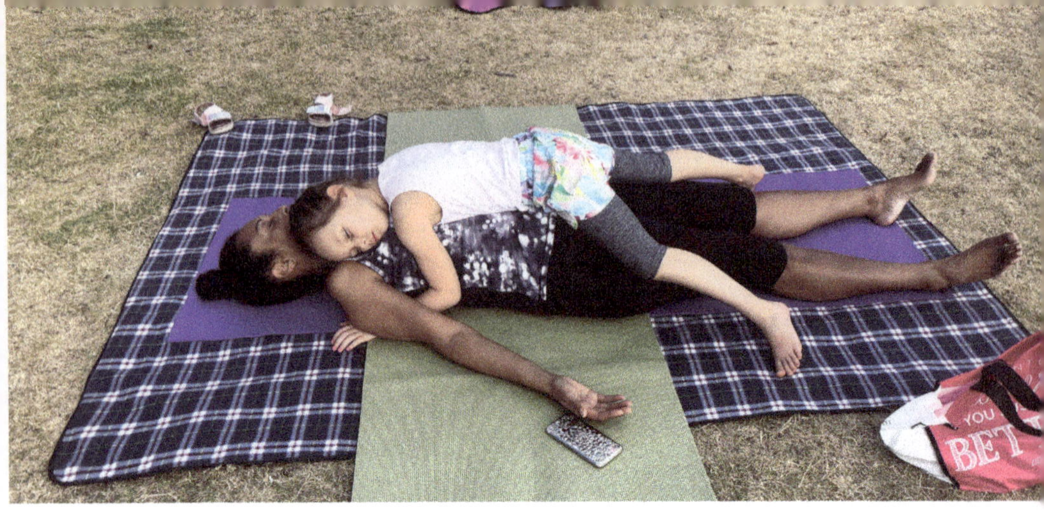

Feel your breath...

Relax scalp, jaw, eyes and eyebrows. Keep focusing on your breath and on letting go. Letting thoughts go, letting tension go, letting expectations go.

At the end of ten–fifteen minutes you will be feeling calm and relaxed. At the end of your meditation, your relaxed state is the perfect time to visualise yourself as healthy, happy and achieving your goals.

When you are ready to come out of your meditation, stretch fingers and toes. Rotate wrists and ankles. Stretch and release your whole body. With a big sigh, release your breath and your body. Roll onto your side and slowly sit up in a comfy cross-legged position.

Continue to breathe for another minute. As you feel the peace grow within you, know that you can take this peace with you as you go about your daily life. Breathe in the energy of peace and success into your life, softly open your eyes and intend to have a wonderful day.

This short relaxation will affect your whole day. You will have more energy, more clarity and more insight than ever before.

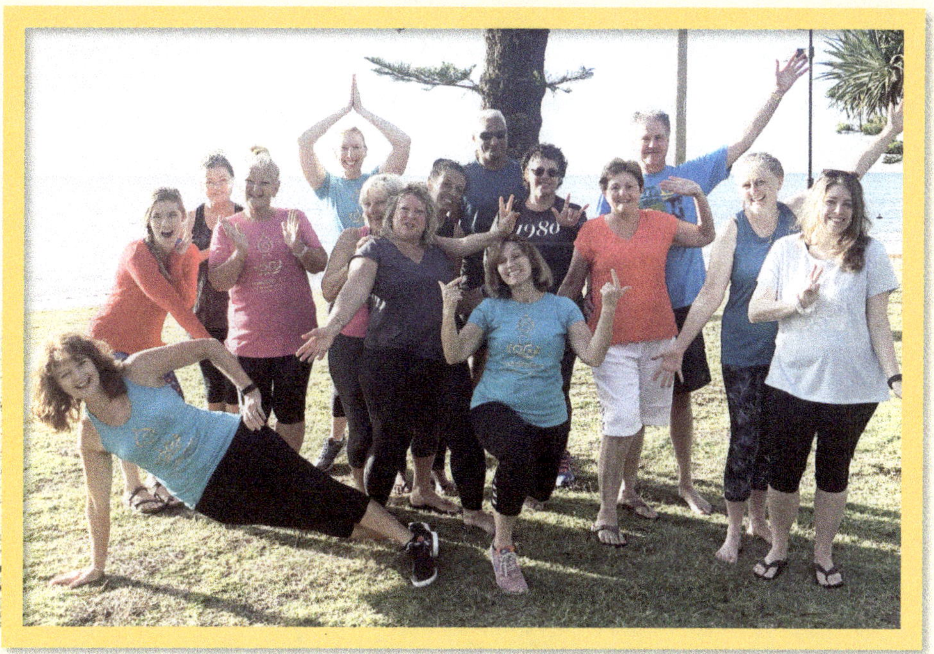

NAMASTE

Namaste means *'the spirit in me acknowledges the spirit in you'*. It is a way of saying *'we are all one'* and that each of us, regardless of who we are or where we come from, deserve love, acceptance and respect.

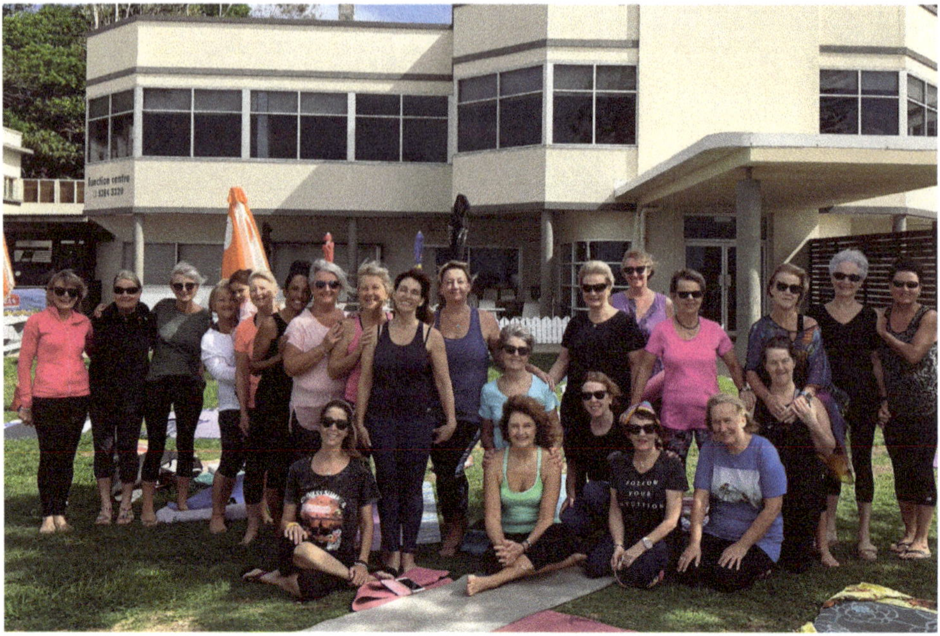

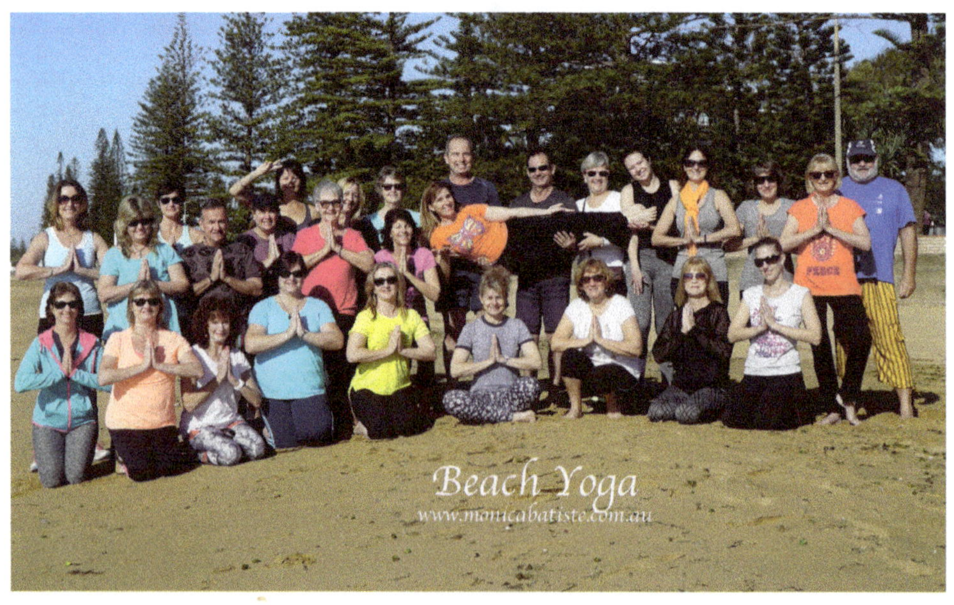

Beach Yoga
www.monicabatiste.com.au

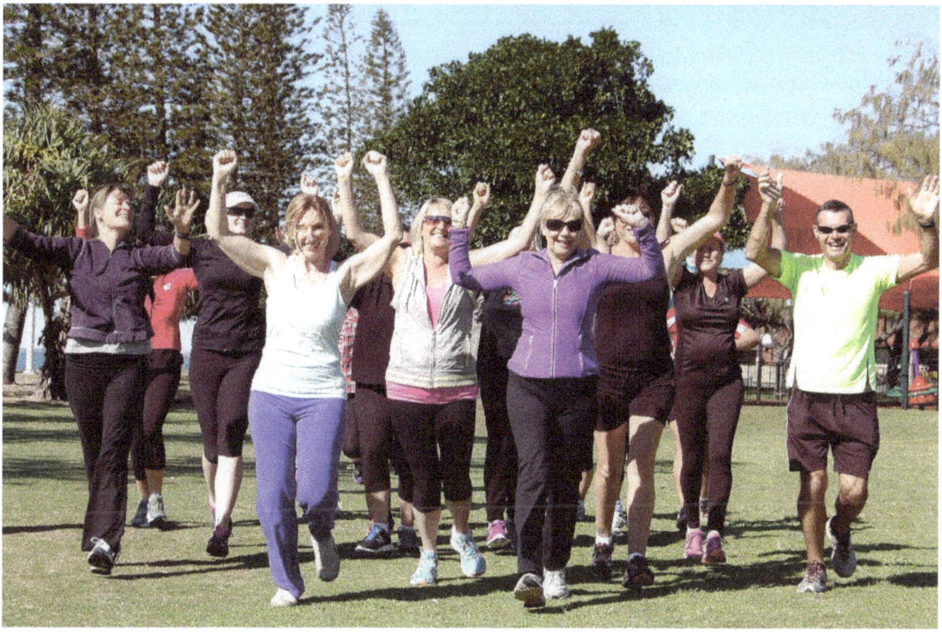

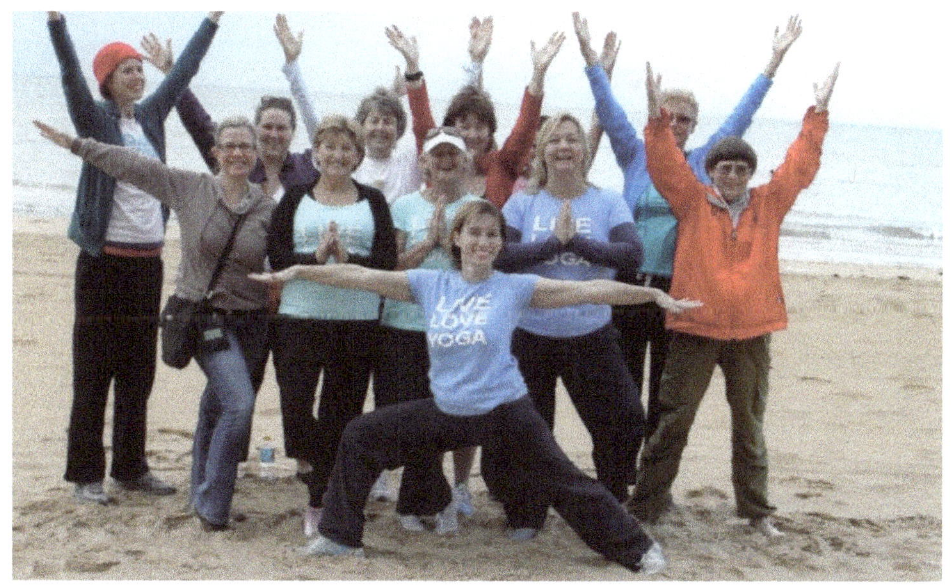

LIVE
LOVE
YOGA

connection

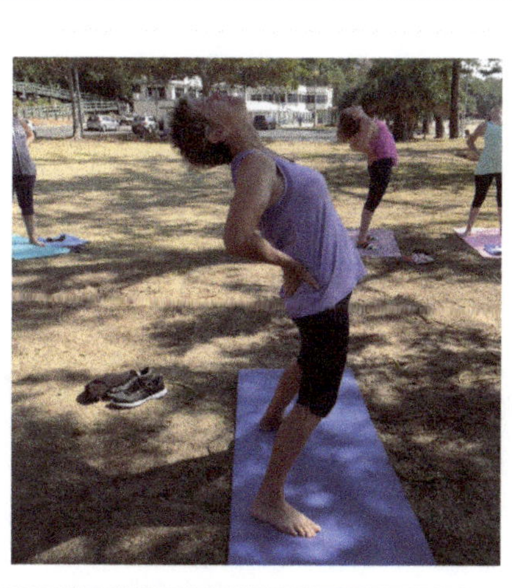

positive
AFFIRMATION

Connection is key

community

positive
AFFIRMATION

Friends are everything

intention

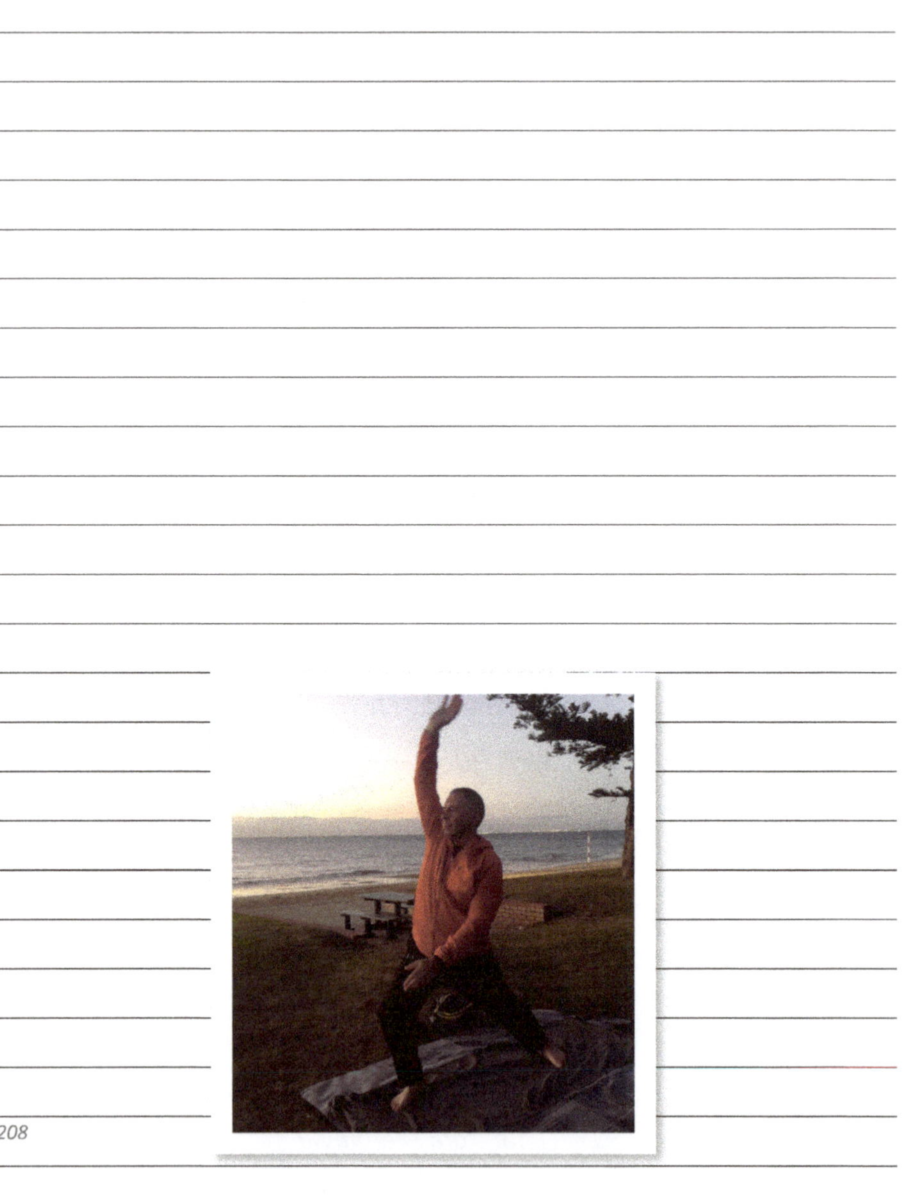

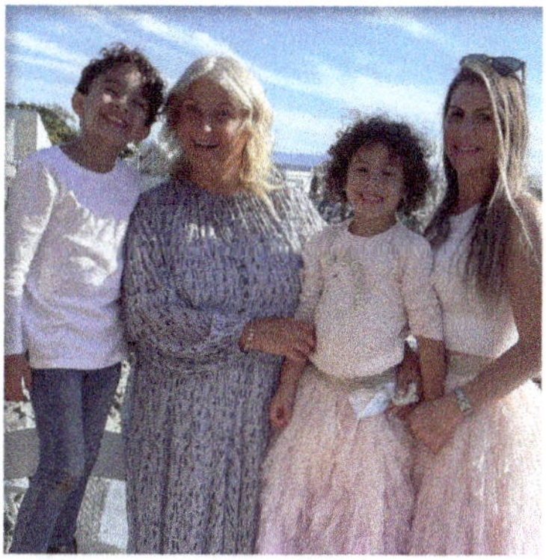

positive
AFFIRMATION

Set your intention

liberty

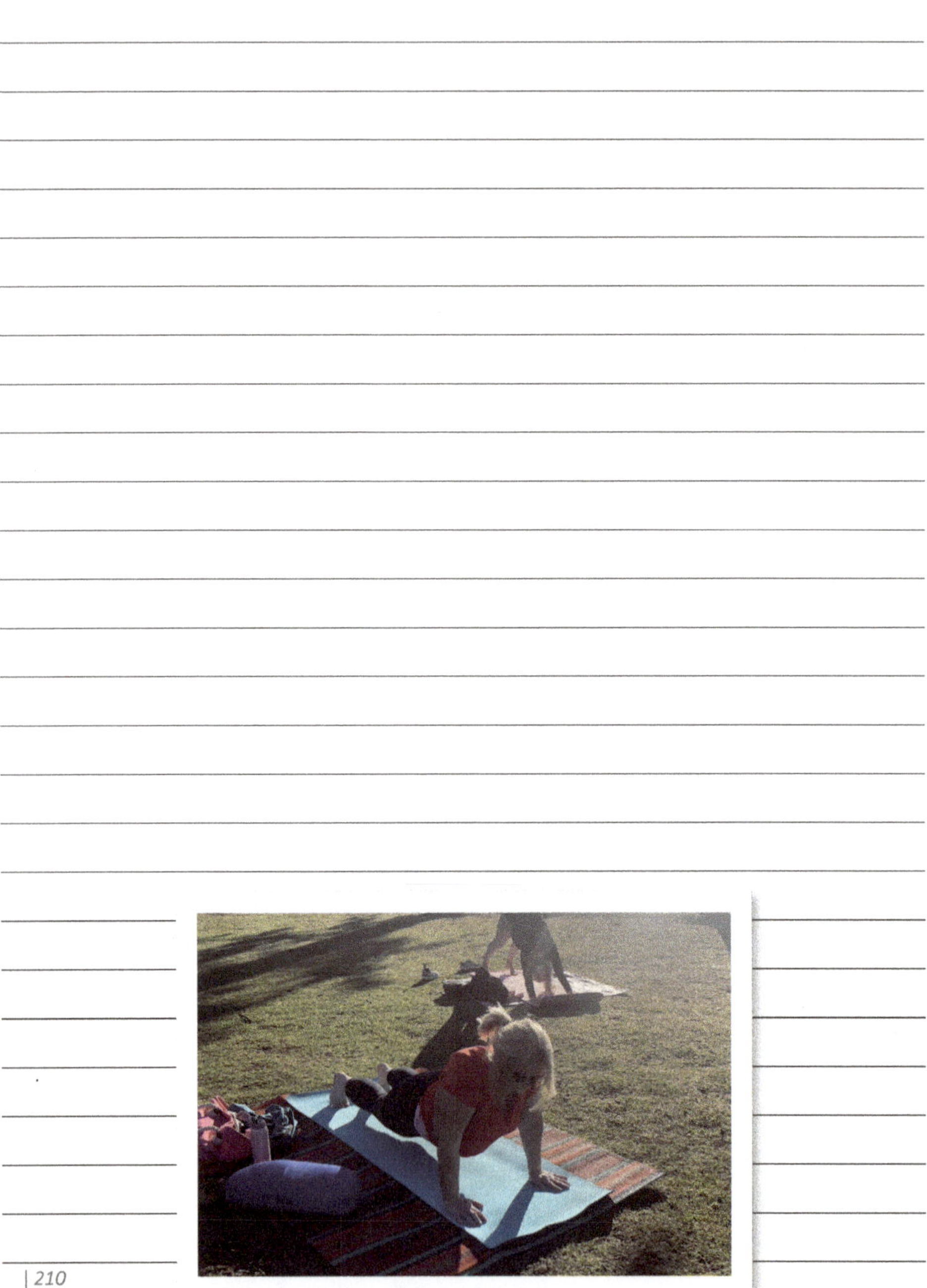

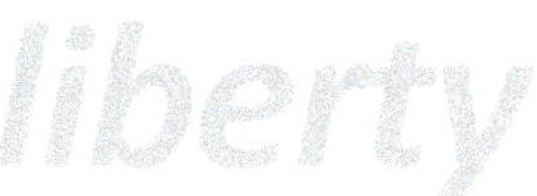

positive
AFFIRMATION

Free to be me

About Monica

My childhood was a mixture of the Aussie battler, German traditions, the military, classical music, drawing, painting, and ballet.

From an early age I was dancing, drawing, reading and painting. Creativity was my link to myself.

My mother was a ballet dancer from Germany, travelling Asia with her troupe when she met my father in Singapore while he was on leave from his tour in Malaysia. My father was a WO11 and did 3 tours with the Australian army, Malaysia, Vietnam, and Korea. When he went to Vietnam I was two years old. He was a kind and funny man, torn by war and PTSD. My mother was in the Dresden bombing of 1945. It was something she would never fully recover from.

My parents married in Singapore 6 months after they met. They had my brother Wayne in Australia in 1961, then returned to Malaysia with the Australian Army from 1961 - 1963 where my sister and I were born. They settled in a war service home in Eastern Creek, Sydney's west, when I was 6 months old.

Eastern Creek was far away from concert halls, art schools and opera houses. My mum opened a ballet school at *Rooty Hill School of Arts* and helped many young girls follow their dreams of being a ballet dancer.

It must have been quite the culture shock for my mother, but we made do with a tape player, an old piano, and a yearly trip to Sydney for the Ballet Eisteddfods. One of my highlights was dancing in the Sydney Opera House when I was 11. I met my best friends at Eastern Creek primary and Rooty Hill high school. It was at Rooty Hill that my art teacher Mr Sullivan 'Boss', taught me to see myself as an artist.

In grade 12, my English teacher Rex Saddler told me I must go to university; something that felt out of my league for a small town girl who didn't believe she could learn. I studied at Universities and Art Colleges. My fragile mental health caused ebbs and flow in my studies. Art was always something I could rely on to bring me to a better place. Because of my love of dance I became a fitness instructor and yoga teacher. I've always loved health and personal development. It's been my greatest privilege to work in this field, with so many beautiful people I am blessed to call friends.

It has been a long drive from that little girl too scared to show her art, too insecure to become a performer, and too small to stand in front – to working on my craft, working on my self-esteem, and making the decision that one day, I would do what I love, and help others do the same.

In love I've had a few starts and stops. I was a single mum with 2 girls when I met Andreas and his two girls. We married 18 months later. We now have seven grandchildren and our family is packed with awesomeoness. He is the greatest supporter of our hopes and dreams.

Thank you Andreas Guetter. I could not have done any of this without you.

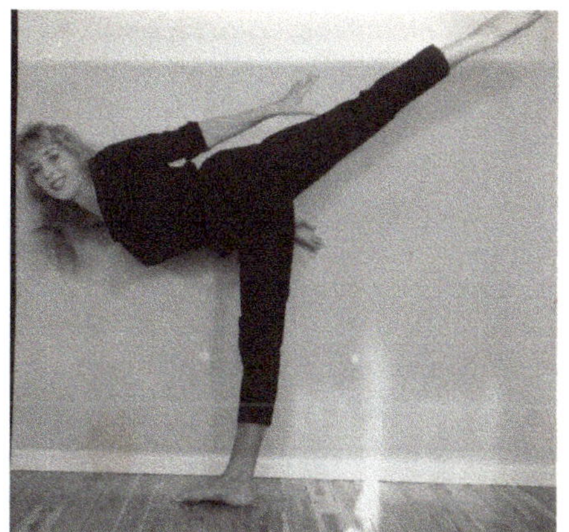

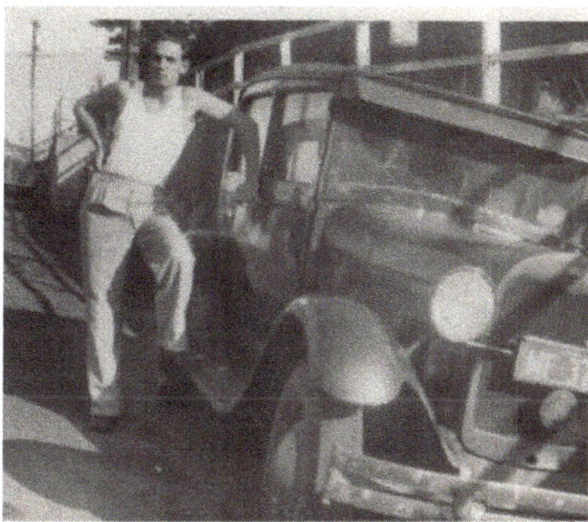

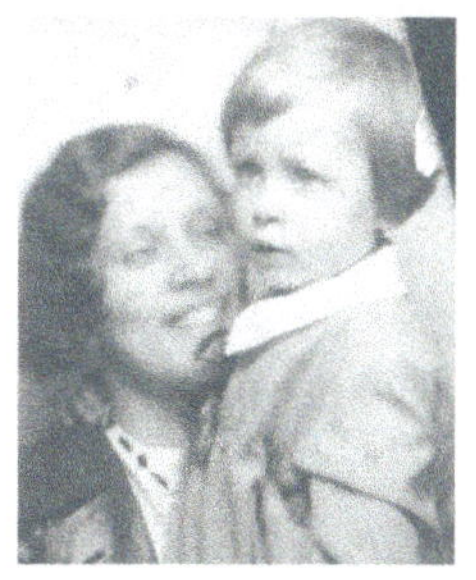

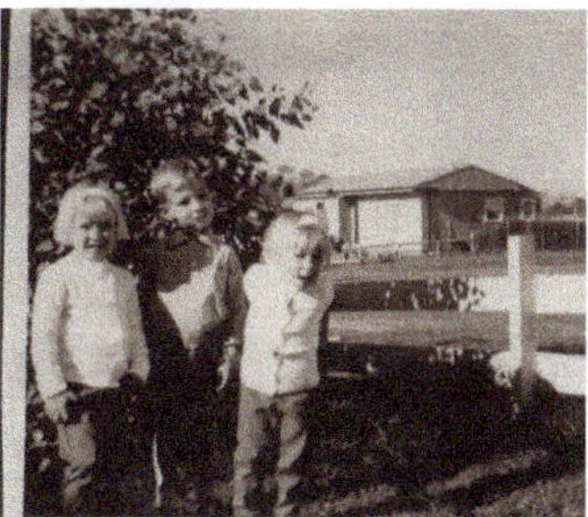

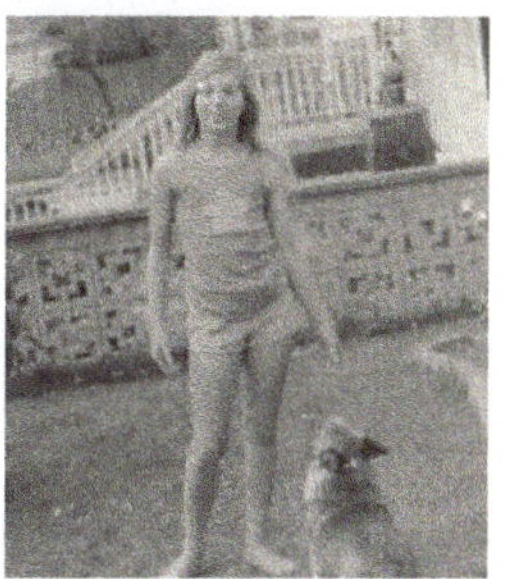

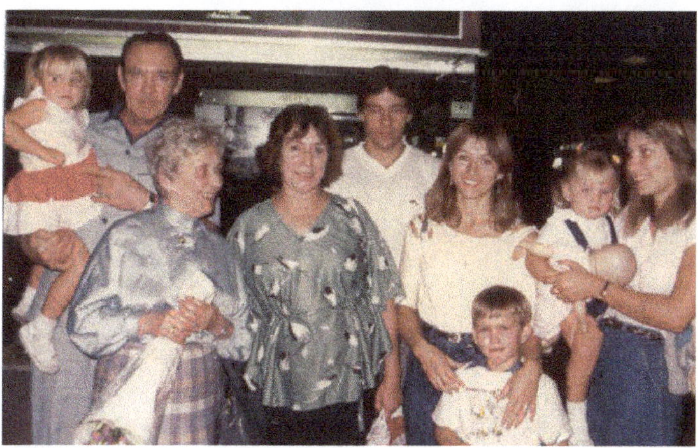

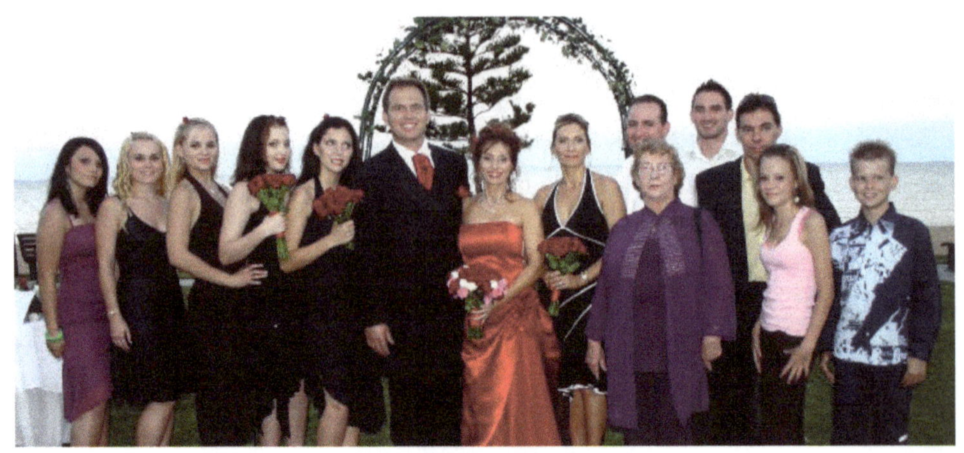

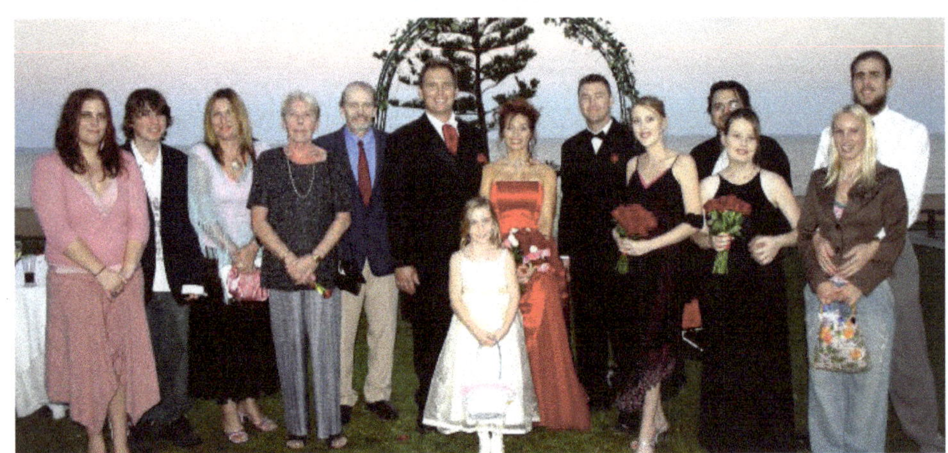

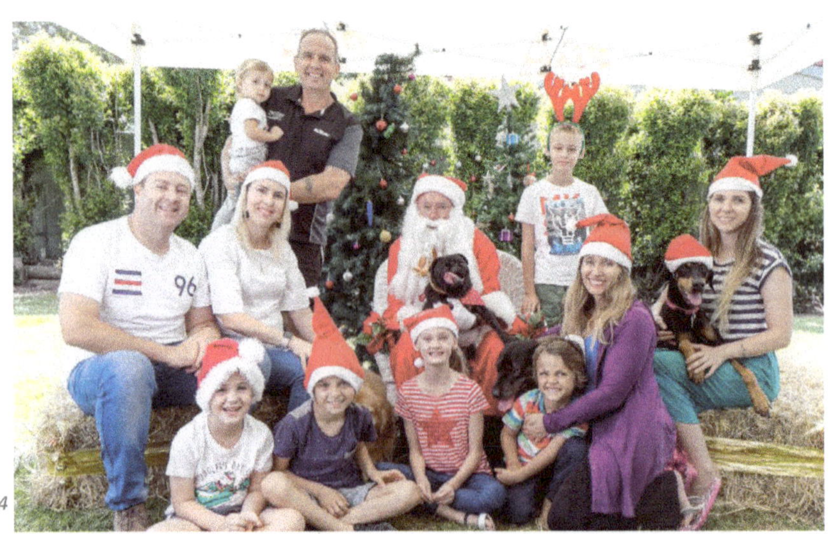

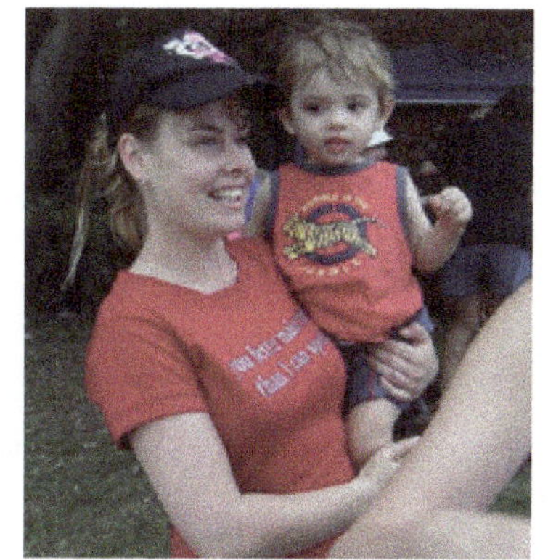

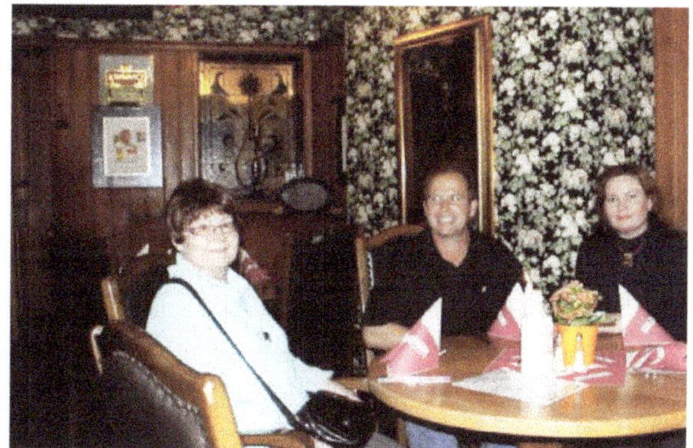

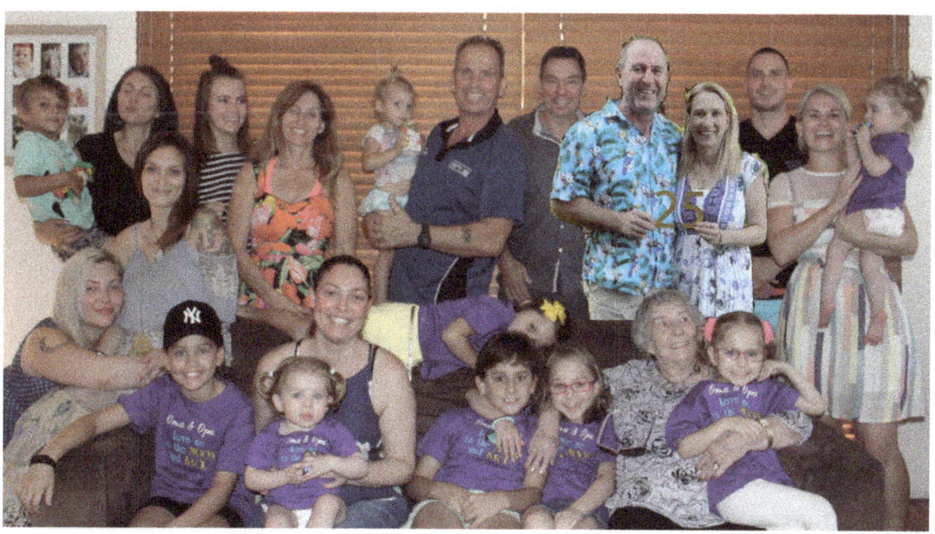

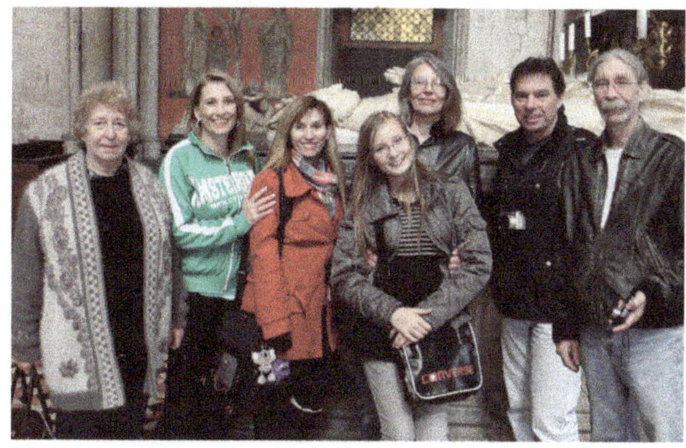

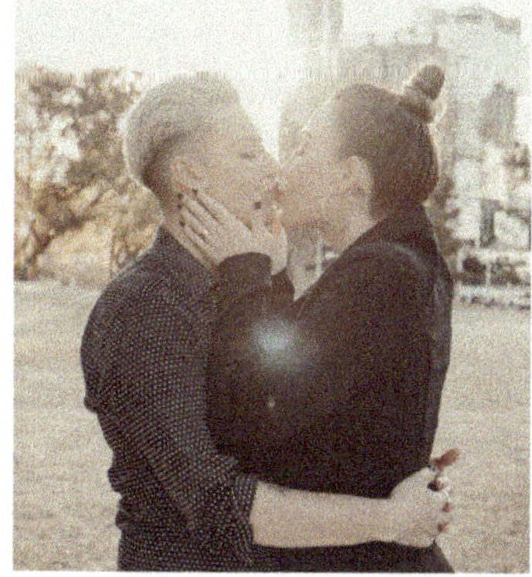

Books and Cards
by Monica Batiste

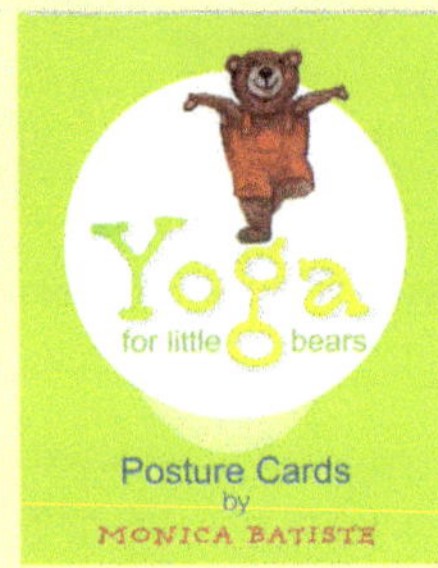
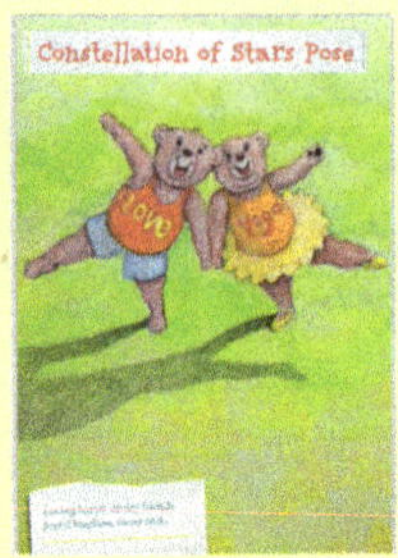
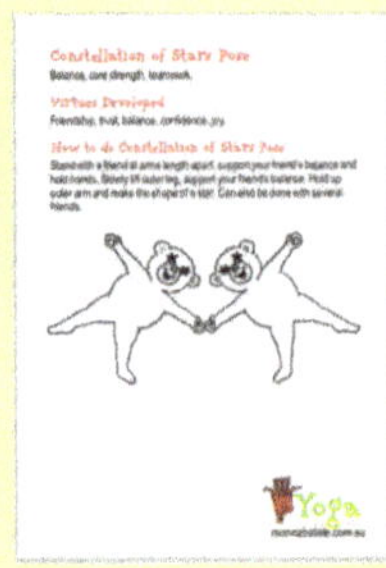
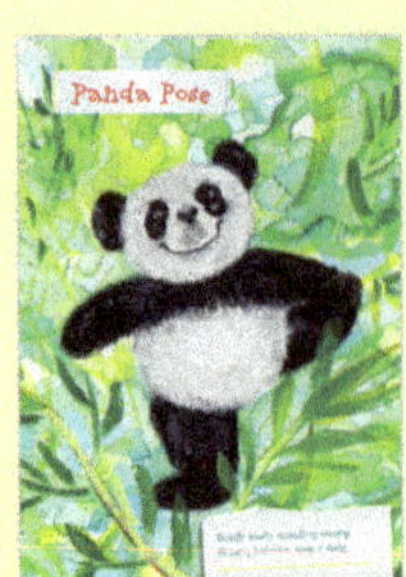

Yoga for little Bears
Posture Cards

Help children grow emotional intelligence through yoga by helping them link movement with emotions.

Our beautifully illustrated deck of 37 cards are the original work of Monica Batiste, who is a yoga teacher, author and artist. Each pack comes in its own magnetic treasure box and each card shows a yoga posture, how to do it, and its benefits.

www.monicabatiste.com.au

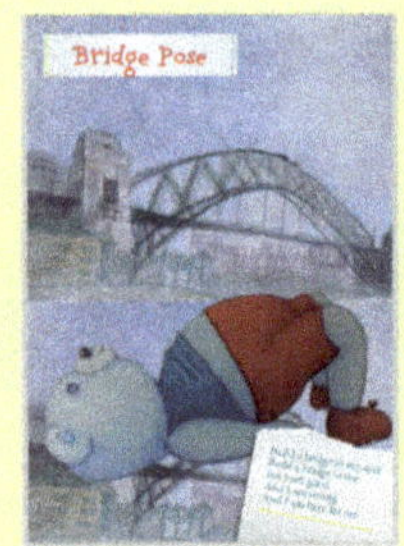
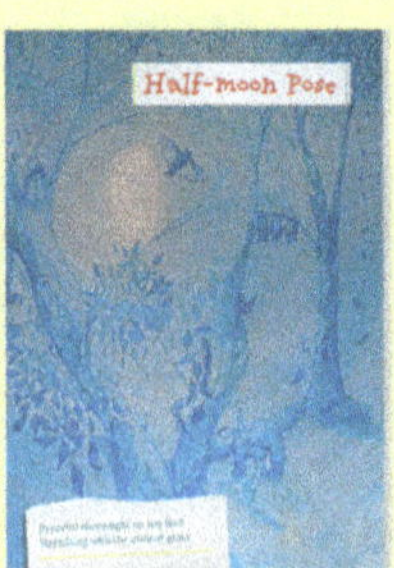
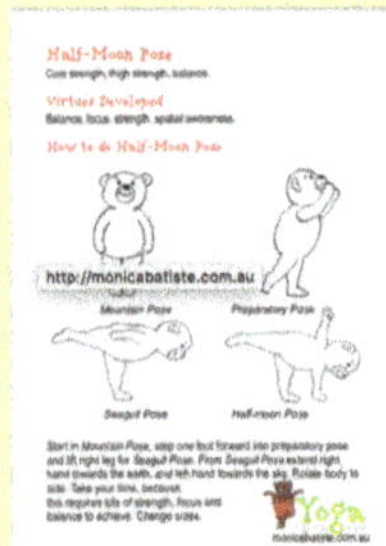
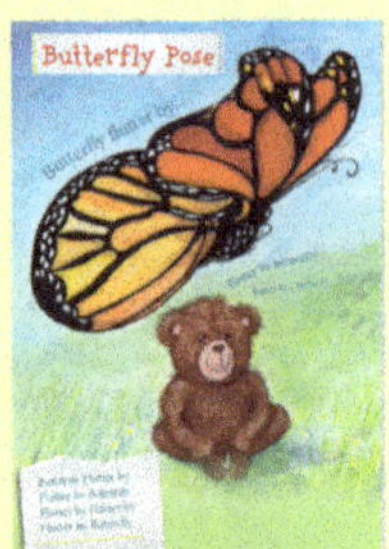

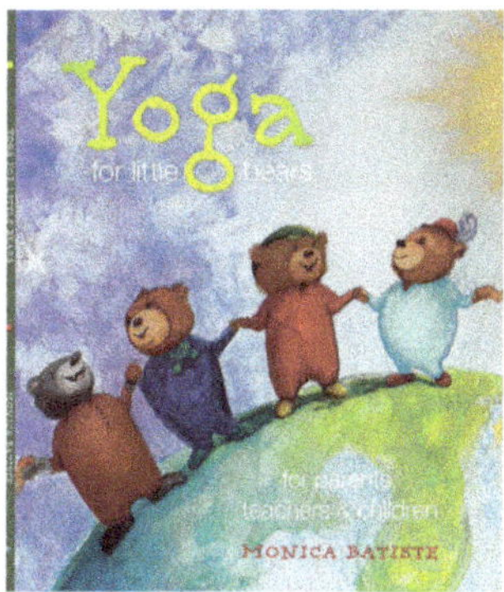

Yoga
for little bears
for parents
teachers & children
MONICA BATISTE

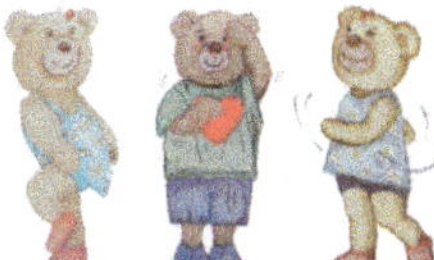

EFT FOR KIDS
EMOTIONAL FREEDOM TECHNIQUE
CALM AND PEACE
MONICA BATISTE

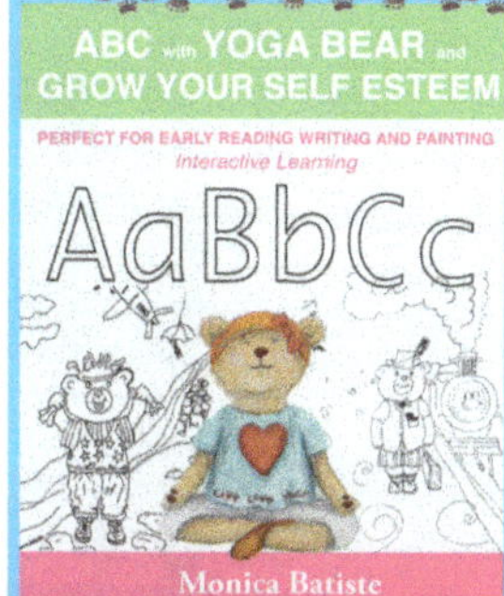

ABC with YOGA BEAR and
GROW YOUR SELF ESTEEM
PERFECT FOR EARLY READING WRITING AND PAINTING
Interactive Learning
AaBbCc
Monica Batiste

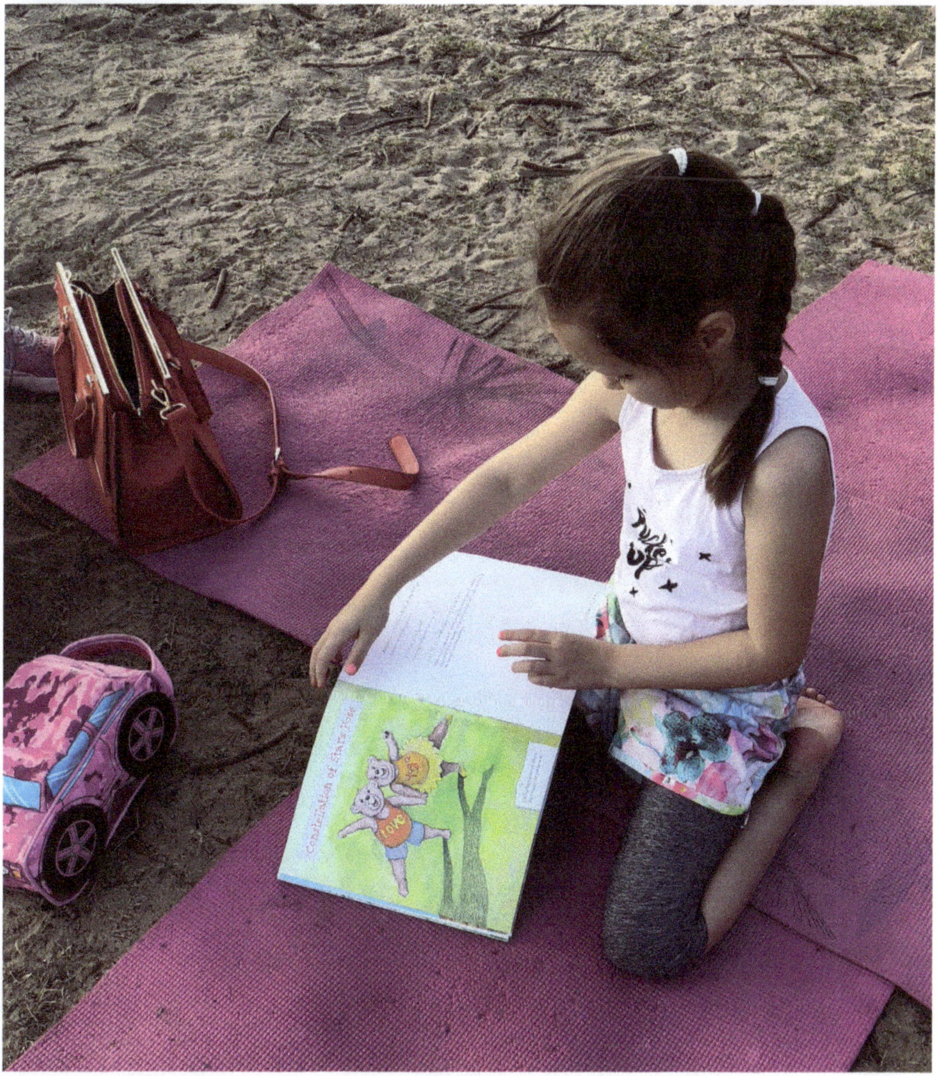

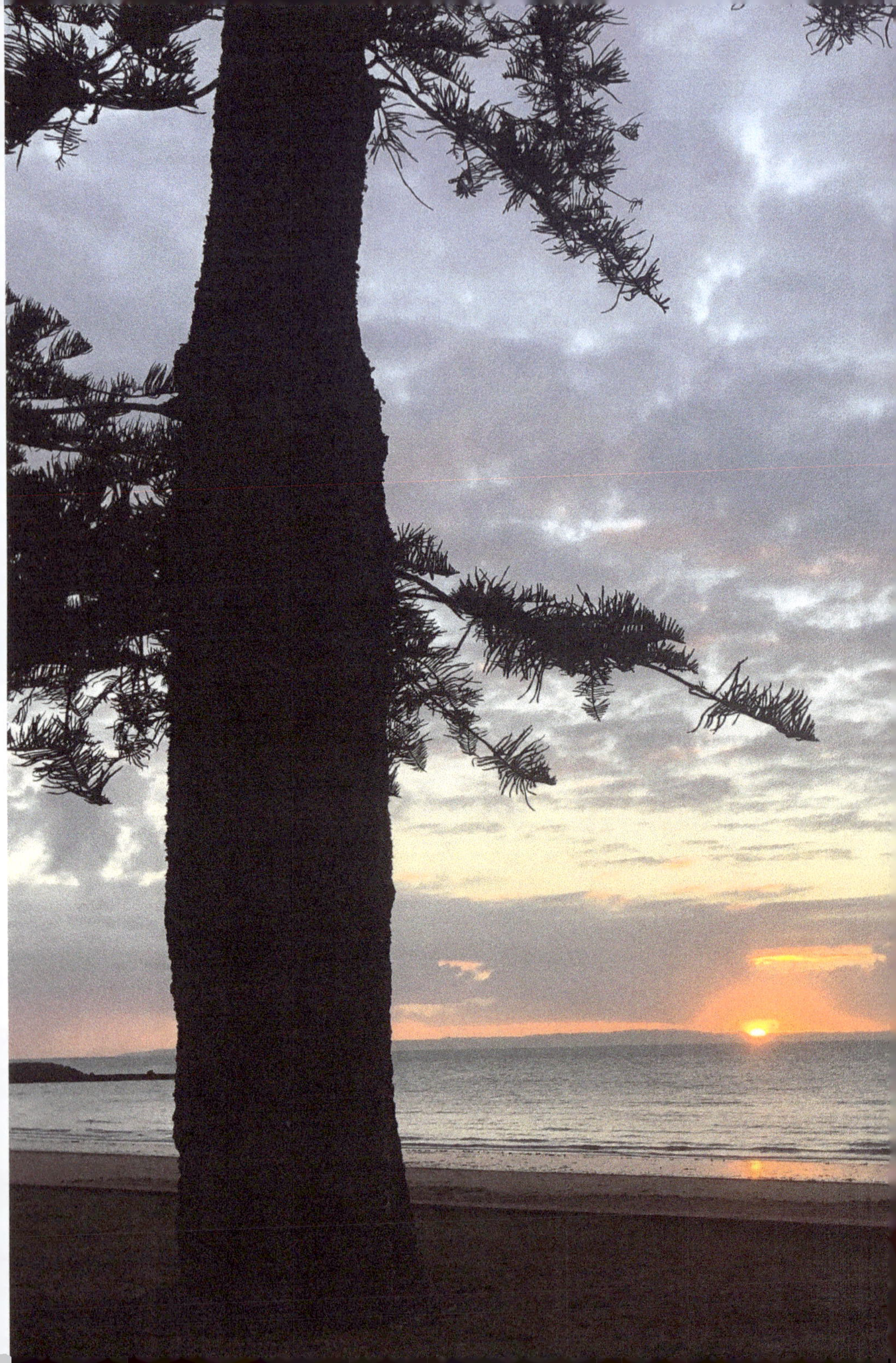

Thank you

Thank you for you. Thank you for your friendship,
thank you for your trust, thank you for your grace and support.
I have learned so much from you, and for this, I am truly grateful.

I know we will continue to learn and grow together
at Suttons beach and around the world.
We've done a yoga retreat in Fiji, the Gold Coast and Chen Rezig.
We have had many birthday celebrations and gatherings.

Keep loving and accepting yourself, just as you are.
Keep opening your heart and hearing the whispers of life.

I wish you all the best for your journey.
We intend to live our best lives.

Monica

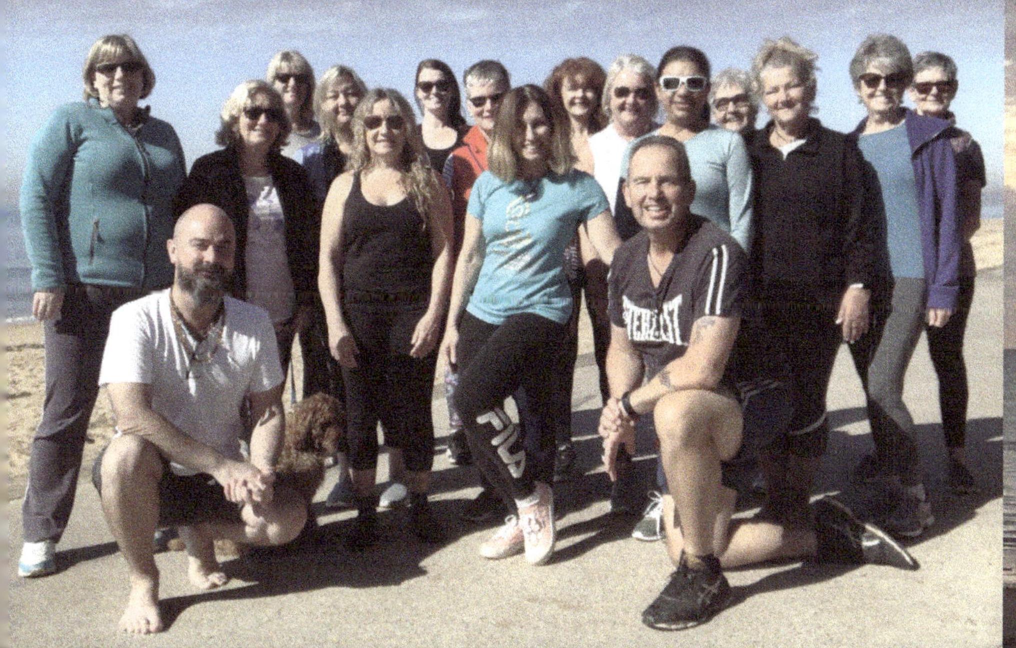

© 2021 by Monica Batiste
Cover photograph and back photo by Elizabeth Wald.
Graphic design by Jane Hayes Watt and Monica Batiste.
Proof read by Friends of Beach Yoga.

Photographers: Chris Dickens, Graeme Collins, Louise Kirk, Fiona Hay, Jacki West, Roger West, Elizabeth Wald, Caroline Watt, Monica and friends from Beach Yoga.

Thank you to Moreton Bay Regional Council for making
Redcliffe such a beautiful and clean place for us to practise
yoga on the beach each morning.

Dedicated to our friends at Beach Yoga. The community and love
we share has given much purpose to our lives. Special thank you to LIsa Parella and
Yolande Cavey for taking care of our class when I'm away. Thank you Lisa Parella for
organising our birthday parties for many years. Thank you Lisa Parella, Louise Devine
and Carmen for helping to organise our Christmas parties.
Thank you to all the beautiful yoga teachers who teach on the Peninsula, and teach
my class while I'm away; Jane Devine, Jeanie Cooper, Sandy Buchan, Shelley Lyons,
Janette Bossevain, Rocky Bossevain, Lisa Lalita Turner, Sam Seghers, Ross Prosser,
Mikhala Batiste, Jo Moore, Verena Bartelsheim, Eileen Hartley, Elly Ellis-Blowers, Guy
Gibson, Amanda Martin, Cate Hando, Andrea Bolding, Lorraine Fudge, Chris Burford,
Beks Thomspon, Areti Le Seur

Thank you Jane Hayes Watt for your graphic design, friendship and creativity.
Thank you to Jamie Palmer for all the love and creativity and friendship we shared.
RIP. You will always be missed.

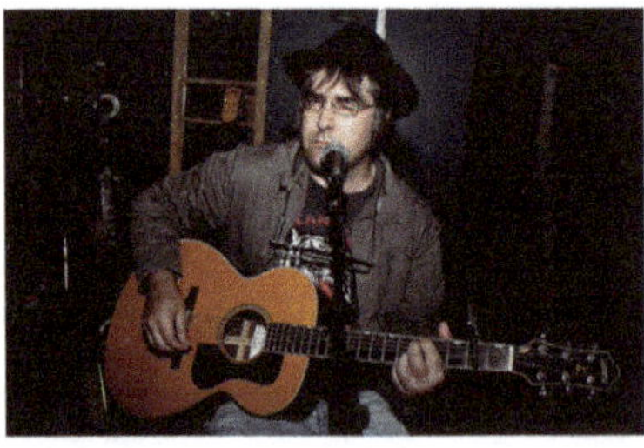
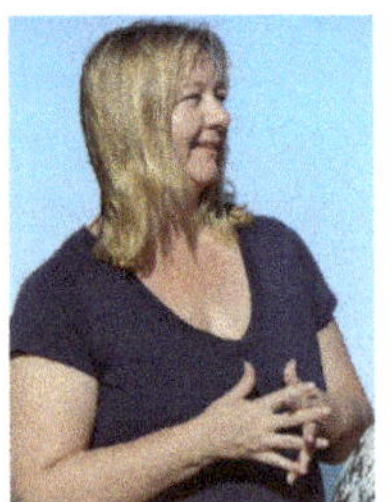

Published by Art & Words Publishing, Margate Queensland
ISBN 9780648373483

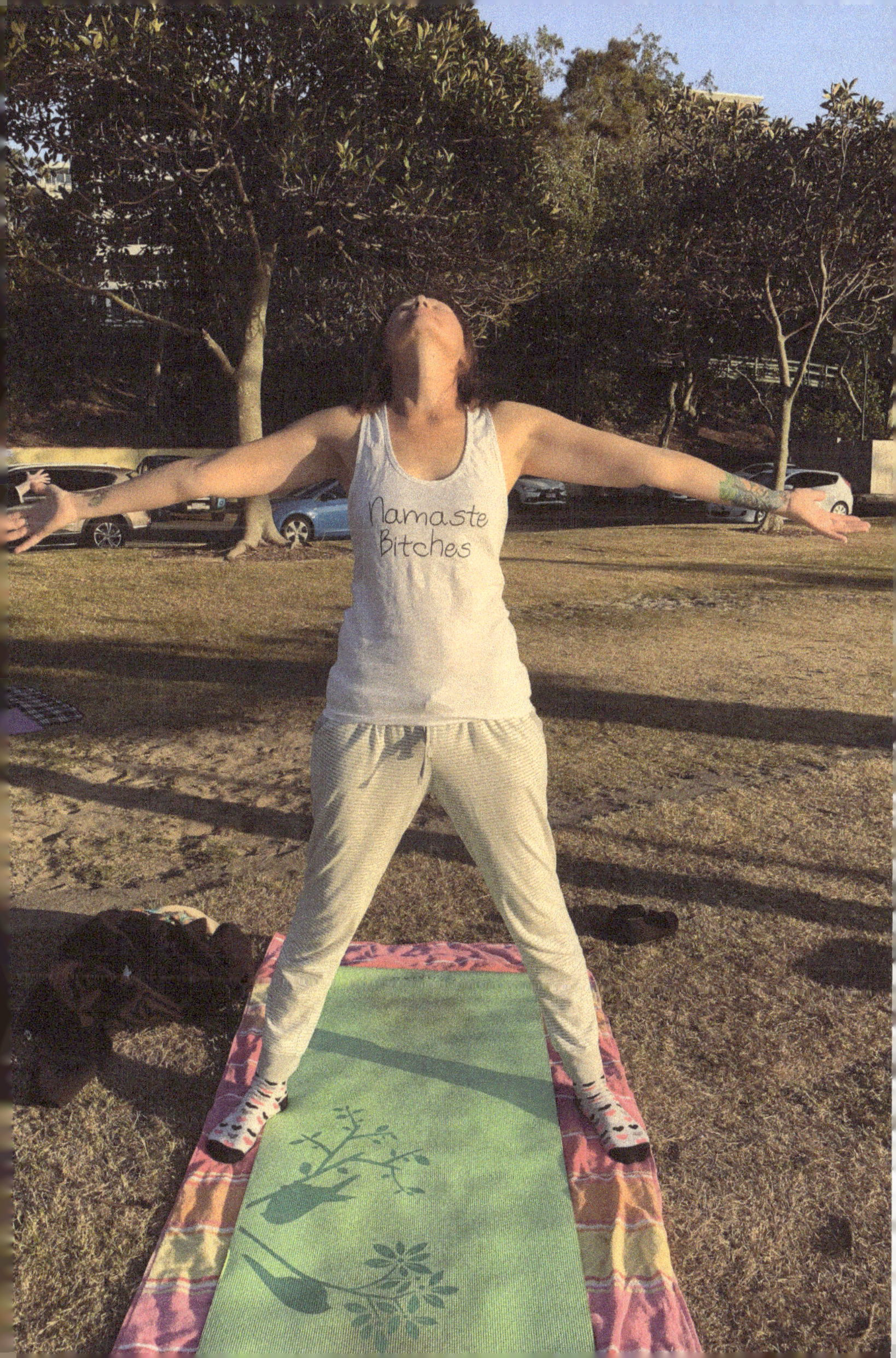
Namaste
Bitches

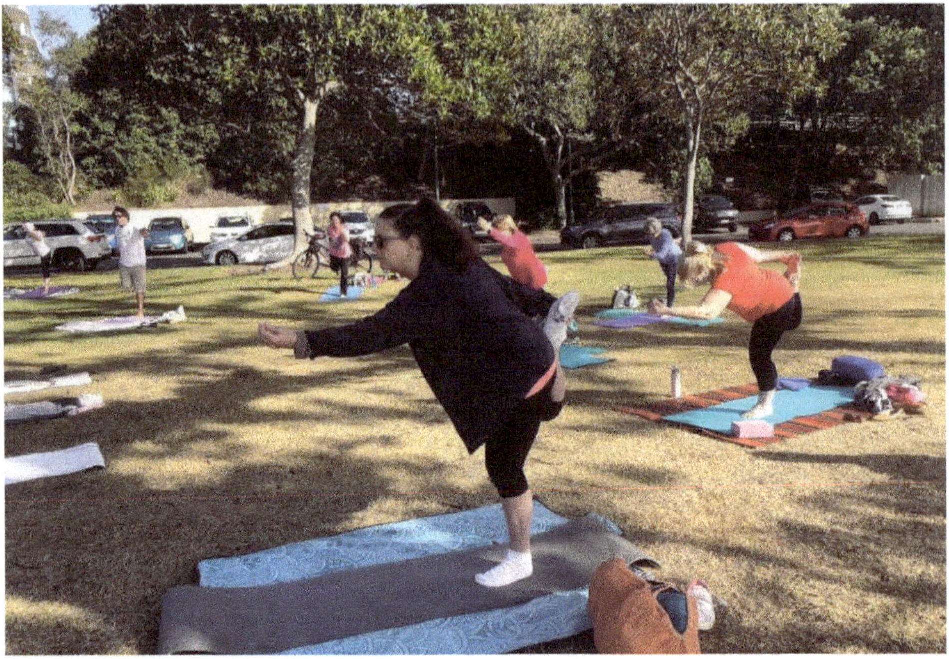

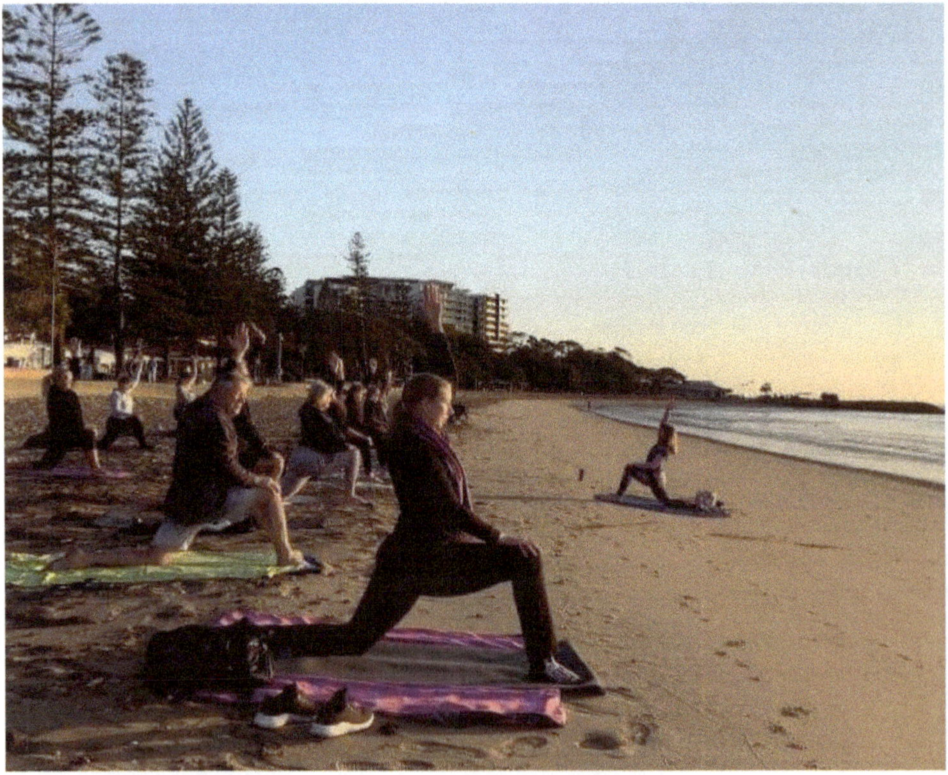

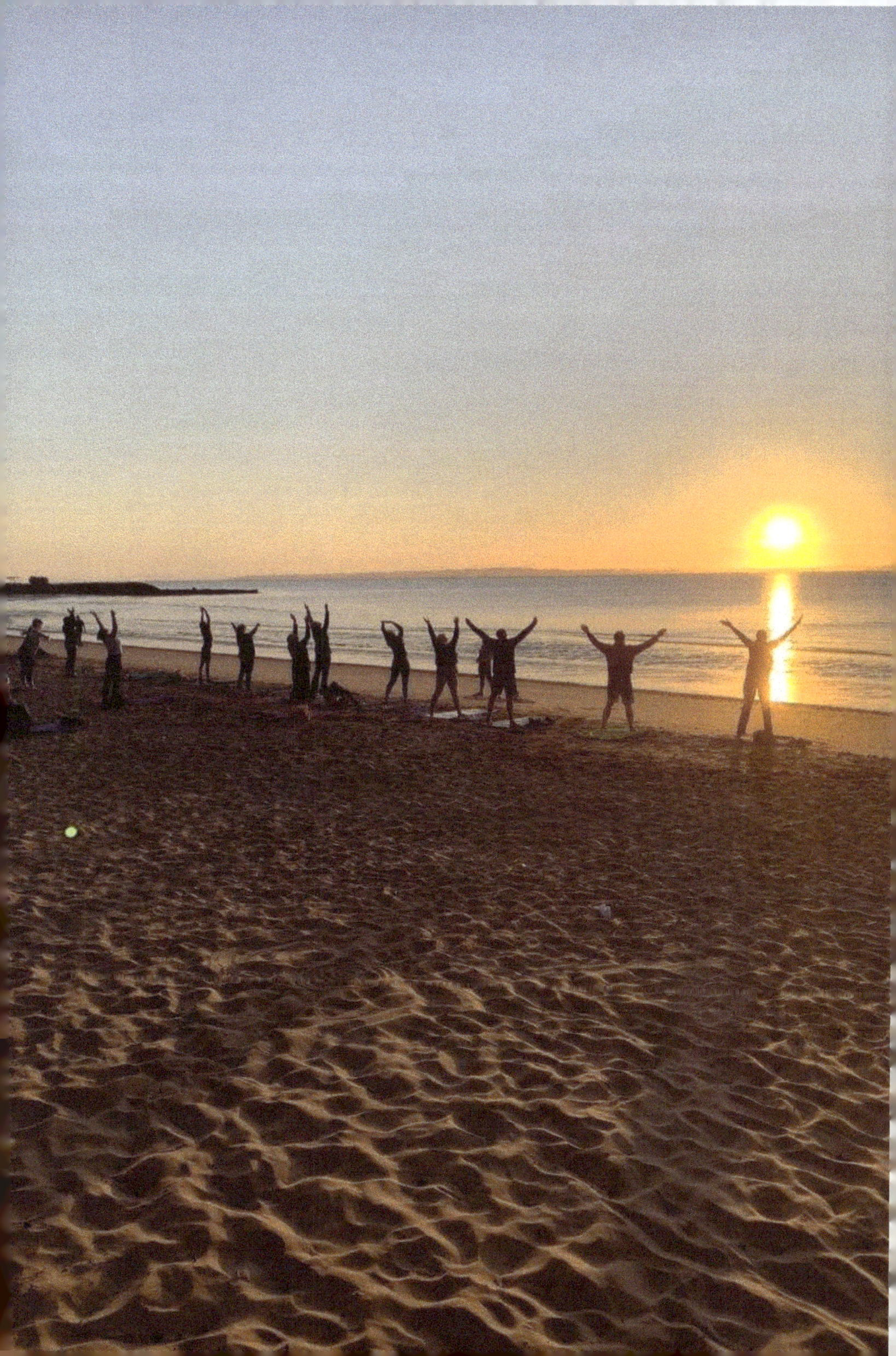

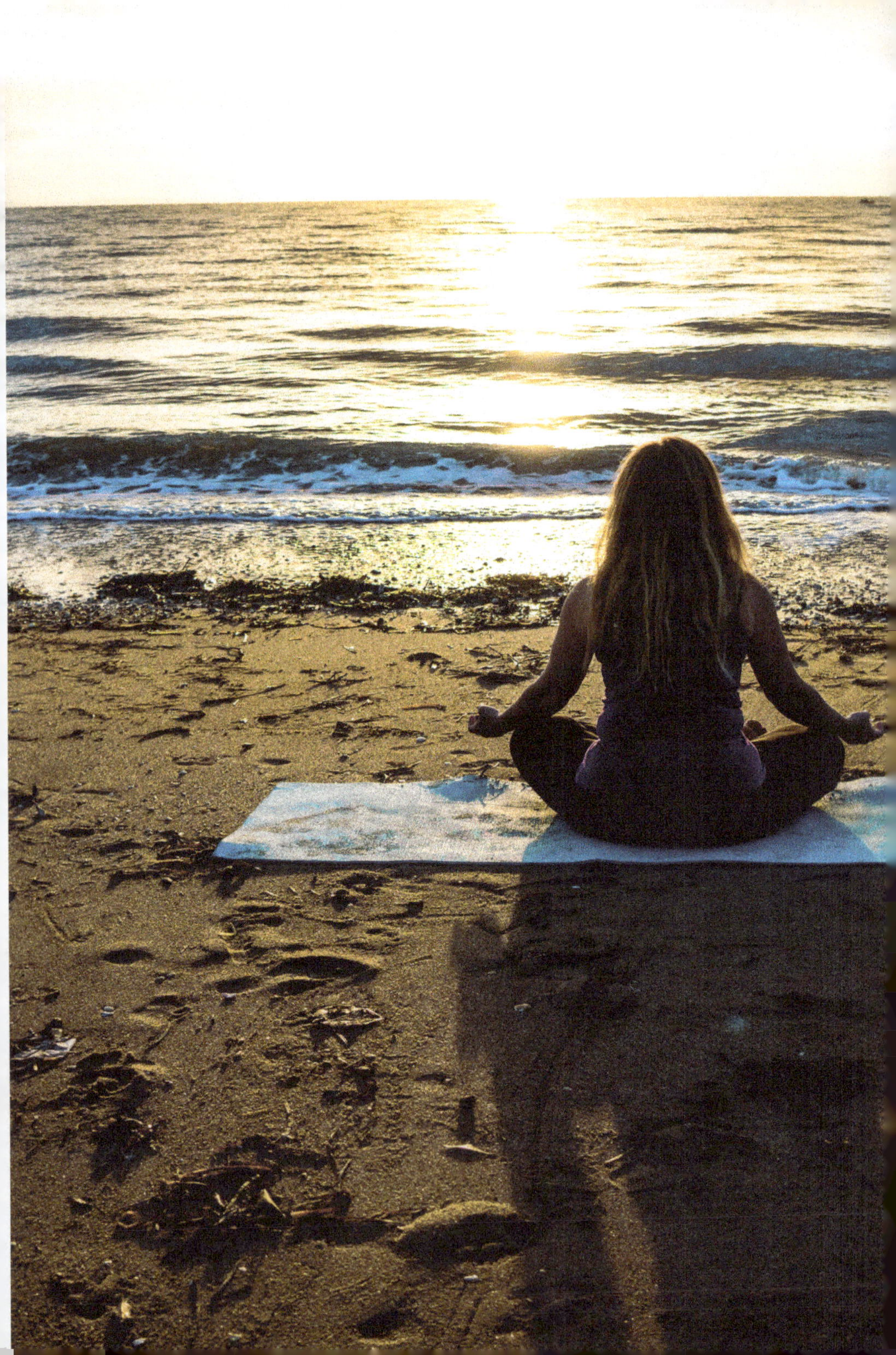

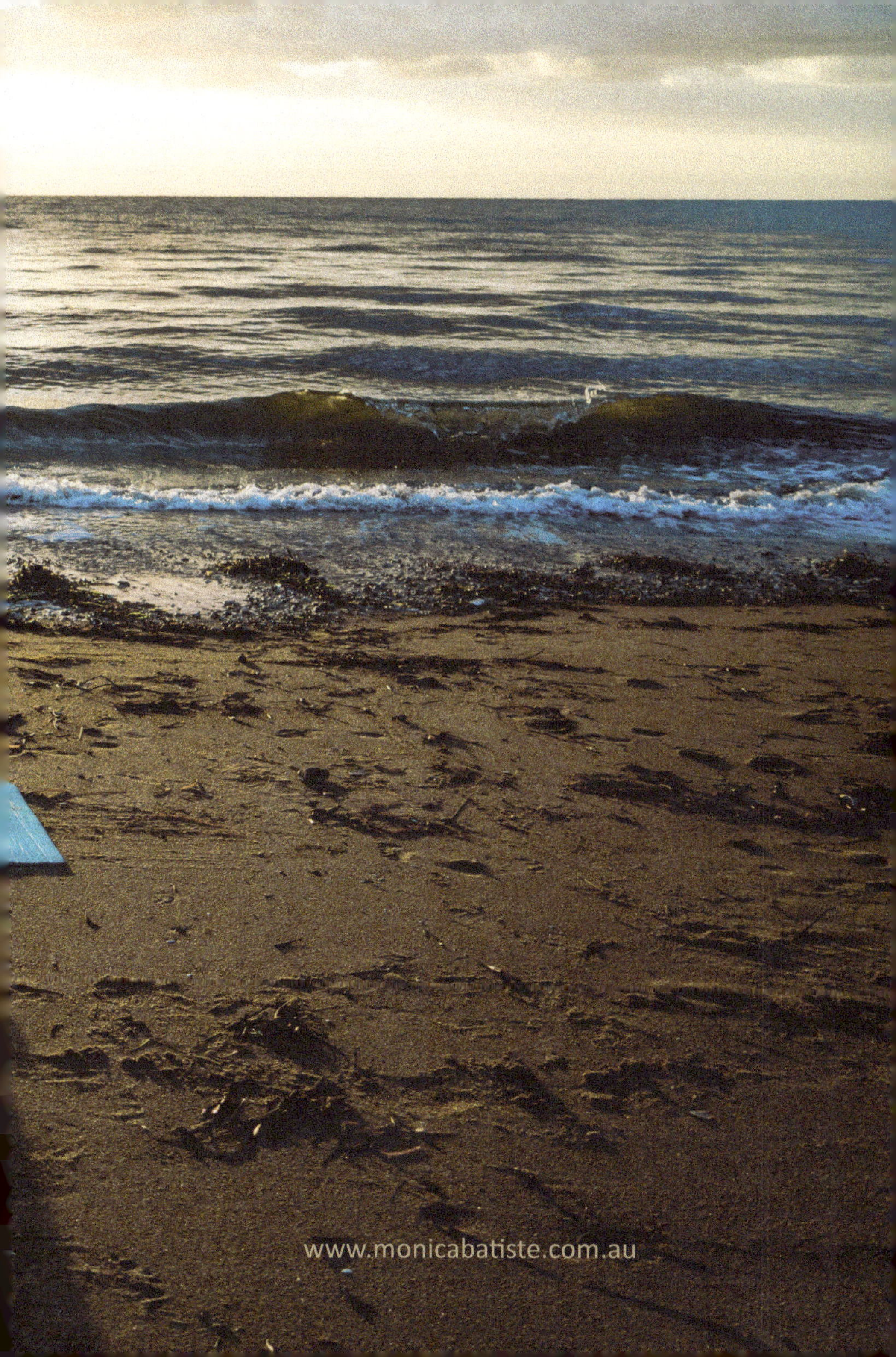
www.monicabatiste.com.au

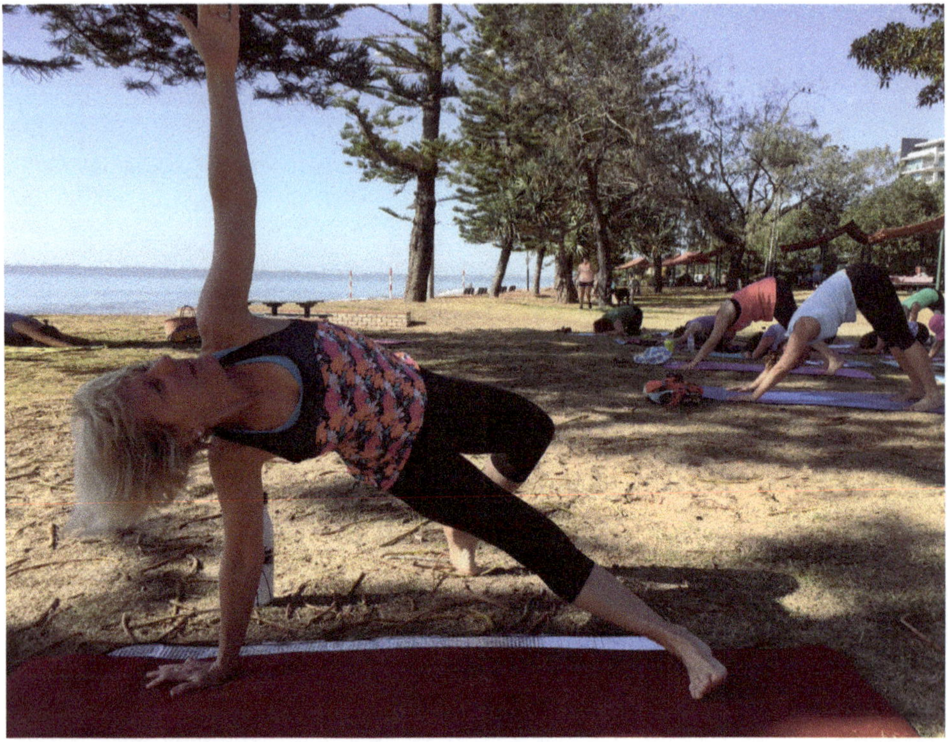

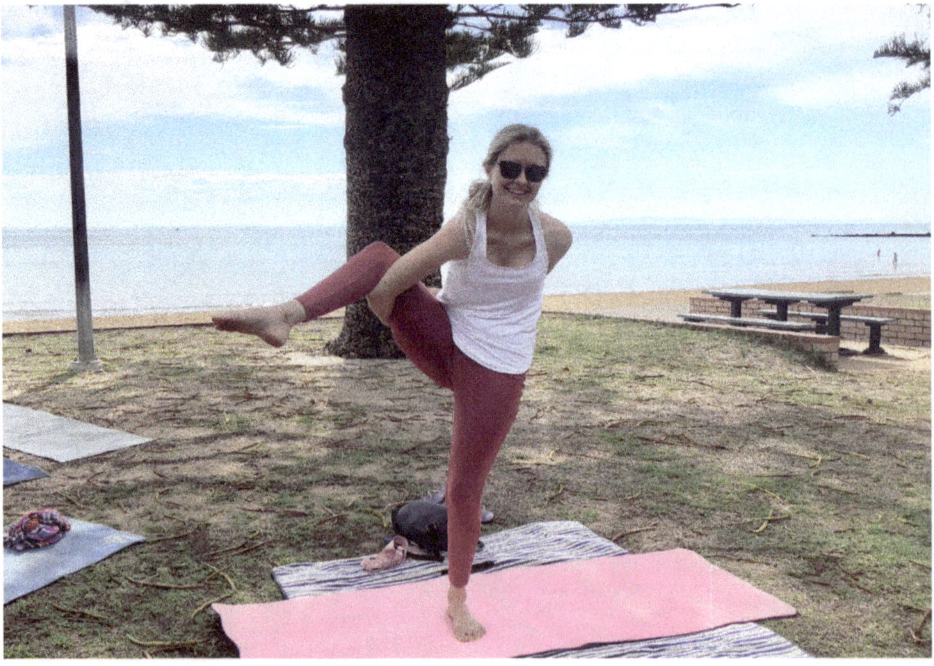